SUPER SKIN

SUPER SKIN

The Doctor's Guide to a Beautiful, Healthy Complexion

Jonathan Zizmor, M.D.
and John Foreman

THOMAS Y. CROWELL COMPANY
New York Established 1834

 Published simultaneously in Canada by Fitzhenry & Whiteside Limited, Toronto.

Designed by Ingrid Beckman

Manufactured in the United States of America

Library of Congress Cataloging in Publication Data

Zizmor, Jonathan.
Super skin.

Includes index.
1. Skin—Care and hygiene. 2. Skin—Diseases.
I. Foreman, John, 1945- joint author.
II. Title.
RL87.Z59 616.5 75-28443
ISBN 0-690-01078-8

1 2 3 4 5 6 7 8 9 10

CONTENTS

INTRODUCTION

Disturbances of the skin, scalp, and hair are a dermatologist's concern, and this automatically puts him into the beauty business. People fear even the most minor ailments because they are disfiguring: thinning hair is more disturbing than a health-threatening infection; a woman's monthly bout of "periodical acne" is more troubling than an ovarian cyst. Dermatology welds people's interest in their health with their even stronger interest in looking good. Because of this unique combination, it is, of all medical specialties, the most interesting to the lay public.

Super Skin addresses readers who have probably read widely but misleadingly in the plethora of popular, but often medically unsound, books and magazine articles on skin maintenance. It's intended for normal people with normal problems, and tells how to avoid or treat the most common skin disturbances (acne, hives, dry or oily skin), how to restore skin if it has been damaged by sun, age, or scarring, and how to protect it from disease. The format may sound familiar but the content is not. Millions of words have been printed about skin, but precious few of these have been based on genuine medical expertise.

Super Skin will address itself not to obscure or crippling skin conditions but to those that trouble nearly everyone from time to time, or those that everybody fears. Acne, for example, isn't limited to teen-agers—probably the majority of women between twenty-five and forty who visit dermatologists are trying to get rid of pimples. Thinning hair, wrinkles, hives, eruptions, dry or oily skin—these are the most common problems that prompt visits to dermatologists. Explaining to the reader how to prevent or deal with such conditions effectively is a recurrent theme throughout these pages.

There's also a section on the benefits of hair transplants for both men and women. It's commonly thought that men lose more hair than women, but this isn't true—nor is it true that transplants work only for men. Actually the technique is equally effective for women.

In the discussion about skin diseases the emphasis is on common diseases or on those that are universally feared. There is a chapter on skin cancer, for example—it's on everybody's mind—but a full treatment of crippling psoriasis isn't offered since it has only a narrow application. Venereal diseases get close attention since they are widespread and, surprisingly, treated by a dermatologist rather than a gynecologist. Dermatology had its historical origins in syphilology, and so it's the skin doctor who knows that three different laboratory procedures are needed before a "positive" response to a syphilis test actually indicates the presence of the disease, or that venereal herpes simplex, which is currently thought of as dangerously serious, is, in fact, rarely so.

Here are a few of the many reasons why popular literature on skin is so often erroneous and misleading: (1) dermatology is too closely linked with cosmetology and cosmetics companies; (2) popular writers who cover the subject don't believe it's necessary to be medically informed; (3) dermatology is of special interest to youth-seekers, who are an especially credulous group; and (4) the recent high degree of interest in "inner ecology" has caused an explosion of fads, fallacies, myths, and misinformation. Vitamin and health-food freaks, and those who promote the products these people buy, either don't know, or don't care, about the damage fad diets can do to skin.

From the beginning, I've wanted this book to be like a visit to the dermatologist. Any clear-thinking layman will be able to read these pages and hopefully learn something that will improve the quality of his or her life. It's amazing how many important questions there are about skin. Birth-control pills, sun exposure, health foods, skin cancers, cosmetics, not to mention the newly glamorous vitamin E—these sorts of things touch on nearly all our lives, and most people haven't got the slightest idea to what ultimate effect. What's worse, the public is so generally misinformed that many of us are unwittingly aggravating skin conditions at the same time we think we're improving them. This is the unfortunate legacy of our culture's "skin mythology," derived and compiled from generations of food fads and corporate cosmetic promotions.

But debunking current myths is only a part of what this book offers.

In general, my bias is candidly positive; I'm bringing the "good news" about skin—and there's plenty of it. These are bona fide glad tidings rather than PR puffery for fad diets or worthless and overpriced cosmetics. Almost every skin ailment is treatable right now, but the reader should be aware of the difference between what is truly helpful and what is bogus consolation. The appearance of youth in anybody's skin can be greatly prolonged. But here again valid dermatological advances are far more relevant than hormone creams, vitamin E oil, diets of kelp, and other faddish flimflam, which at the very best have only a placebo effect.

Chapter 1

Untold Truths About Skin Care

I'd like you to take the following short True-False test to see how much you already know about skin care.

Athlete's foot is catching............True____False____
Moisturizing lotions are my best
protection against dryness ....True____False____
The pH factor of what I put
on my skin really matters.........True____False____
Eating health foods will
improve my complexion ....True____False____
Hypoallergenic makeup provides
needed protection for my
skin...True____False____
Women never go bald................True____False____
Birth-control pills are bad
for my skin ....True____False____
Eating chocolate can give me
pimples ....True____False____
Skin cancer is a life-
threatening disease ....True____False____

Positive syphilis tests
never lie.................................True____False____

First exposure to poison ivy
causes the worst case ever.........True____False____

Massaging the scalp promotes
hair growth................................True____False____

I can get venereal disease
from a toilet seat........................True____False____

These questions embody only a selection of the myths surrounding skin care. There's hardly another topic so confused by misinformation and public misconceptions. If you haven't guessed already, every one of the statements above is false, except for the last one. Yes, you can get a type of VD from a toilet seat, specifically a condition called scabies (fleshy, itching papules on the waist, wrists, and genitals). The fact that most people think all the other answers are true too is a measure of how confused everybody is!

In the chapters that follow, I'm going to explain the answers to all these questions, tell you which diseases are contagious and which aren't, those cosmetics to depend upon and the ones to avoid, what causes acne and why, and so on. My desire in this chapter is to provide a simple description of the skin and to tell you the best basic care regimen for your own.

The way you look depends on how healthy your skin is. And many skin problems are due to nothing more than a lack of understanding of the skin and the forces that affect it. Your skin is basically divided into two compartments. The protective epidermis is on top; it's separated from the nourishing dermis below by what's called the basement membrane. As you read this page, the bottom layer of your epidermis is rapidly manufacturing new cells. They'll make their debut on the surface of your flesh as soon as the intervening layers are rubbed, washed, burned, or scaled away. The normal transit from the basement membrane to surface level is 364 hours, a shade over fifteen days.

These cells start life swollen with moisture, gradually flattening as they progress toward the surface. Many skin diseases are related to this transit schedule. For instance, the "heartbreak of psoriasis" (that awful scaling of the skin) witnesses cells that have a transit ten times the normal speed. Dandruff is another case of too-rapid cell transit and is really just mild psoriasis of the scalp. The epidermis is primarily a protective layer against the world. Most of the skin's chemical work is done in the dermis, with one major exception: the melanocytes. These are the cells that produce the protein melanin that gives skin its pigment.

The dermis is a completely different matter. It is packed with appendages such as oil glands, hair follicles, blood vessels, nerve tissue, sweat glands, and such exotica as fibroblasts. These latter, when you're under stress, may turn magically into entities called histiocytes, which are first-line defenders against the intrusion of any foreign matter. Fibroblasts also may (or may not, it's an open question) produce collagen, a protein that is the major building block of the dermis. Collagen and elastin, another protein substance, give the skin its tone and suppleness.

The dermis is intimately involved with the bloodstream since the blood vessels that feed the skin are located there. The capillaries in the dermis carry more than just food. They are the conduits for acnegenic (acne-causing) and pustular-causing medicines and substances, whose symptoms begin in the dermis.

Taken together, the dermis and epidermis do not form a simple web. Each part of the body has its own requirements vis-à-vis oil glands, nerve sensors, and so on, so the overall composition of the skin varies considerably from nose to knee. On the other hand, any successful skin care program must individually consider both compartments and their separate needs and reactions.

You look the way you do (complexion-wise) for several not-very-mysterious reasons. For instance, genetics. If your mother had acne, you probably do too. The same goes for more serious things like skin cancer. This is summed up in a concept called "end organ sensitivity." In the case of acne, the end organ whose sensitivity matters is the oil gland. If yours are too sensitive to whatever's in your bloodstream, they will be stimulated to excessive oil production. Result: a high incidence of oil occlusion (clogged pores) and attendant acne. Another person with a lower end organ sensitivity level could tolerate the same blood level of hormones or acnegenic substances and not produce excess oil or have acne.

Besides genetics, the climate in which you live will play a big part in the way you look. People who live in warm places inevitably get much more sun exposure. Fair-haired, blue-eyed people living in tropical environments, like many Australians, have a higher incidence of sun-related diseases such as skin cancer and malignant melanoma (dark blotching).

Often your occupation or life-style might bring you into unusual contact with weather, water, or chemicals. These things plus the detergents, cosmetics, and soaps of daily living all help determine your appearance. In most cases though, the overall quality of your life plays the biggest part. Increased sex, humorously held to be a sure cure for acne, usually accompanies a more easeful and relaxed life. Sex itself doesn't cure pimples, but as your overall life improves, so will the quality of your skin.

Even though every one of us has our own individual

tolerance levels and susceptibilities, we can all be said to fall into one of the three following skin categories: oily, dry, and normal. How each of us can best improve our skin is determined by, first, accurately diagnosing ourselves. Look in the mirror, and consider. Acne, for example, is a clear signal of over-oiliness, particularly if it's seasonal. The classic syndrome is acne in the winter that clears up in the summer. The clear-up is often due to sun exposure, which encourages peeling. The peeling takes off the oil plugs that clog the oil glands along with the top layer of skin. And when the pores are opened, the risk of inflammation by trapped fatty acids is dramatically reduced.

You can give yourself a simple test for oiliness. In the morning, before washing or showering, wipe a strip of brown paper of the sort used in supermarket bags back and forth across your forehead. If there's enough sebaceous oil on your skin to make the paper translucent, you could be too oily.

Perhaps you suffer from winter itch (xerosis, in medical parlance), that condition of rashes worse in the creases of elbows, knees, and eyes. Perhaps you just suffer from uncomfortable dryness or get little dry patches on your body. These are common symptoms of skin that's unnaturally dry.

What's important here is to understand that proper care of the skin rests on choosing between distinctly different daily skin care regimens for each type of epidermis, with appropriate recommendations on soaps, astringents, shampoos (since hair condition and complexion are affected by the same factors), and cosmetics. After that, there's a short discussion of helpful hints on care of the dermis.

A Regimen for Oily Skin

SOAPS

If you're oily, the more you wash the better. Three times daily is the minimum, preferably after each meal. Your goal is to degrease the skin, which will alleviate the acne that stems from too much oil. Mildly oily skin reacts very well to Ivory soap. There are numerous over-the-counter (OTC) acne soaps for tougher oil problems, among them SAStid, Sulphur Soap, Acnaveen, and Acne-Aid. These contain strong drying agents and/or substances that promote peeling, such as sulfur and resorcinol. If you're black or dark complexioned, beware of resorcinol; it can cause dark stains and blotches on your skin. And if you're using one of the acne soaps, start slowly. You don't want to dry out or start peeling too fast; wash once daily at first and gradually increase to two or three times a day.

ASTRINGENTS

Astringents are degreasing agents that clean off the skin. They are vigorously recommended for oily-skinned people, and your pharmacist can make you a good inexpensive one. It's called 2 percent salicylic acid tincture. If you purchase a prepared astringent look for one that contains alcohol. Seba-Nil is a good brand, and it comes packaged in small bottles as well as towelettes, both convenient for people who need continued applications. Most astringents are predominantly alcohol, and a modest bottle of rubbing (isopropyl) alcohol will do as well as most expensive alcohol-based products. Acetone products are dramatically good; your skin might not have felt so clean in years as after an astringent application.

SHAMPOOS

It's impossible to effectively treat oily-skinned acne without considering the oily hair that's above it. Unless the hair is unusually thin or damaged, I advise a strong detergent (alkaline) shampoo that rids the hair of grease and oil. Some shampoos, such as Pernox, Zetar, and Zincon, are formulated specifically for acne-oily people. Buy more than one brand, since a common problem with these products is that they work well for a week or so, then seem to stop. The reasons lie in our individual reactions to the active ingredients. So, if Zincon, whose active ingredient is zinc pyrithione, mysteriously stops working, perhaps you should switch to Zetar, whose active ingredient is tar.

Shampoo daily, but don't overdo it with the acne shampoos. Like acne soaps, they contain strong degreasers to which you must give your skin time to acclimate. Most products contain either tar (derived from petrochemicals, coal, or pine) or salicylic acid. Just as good as the previously mentioned shampoos are Head & Shoulders, Sebulex, Sebutone, plus any of the acne or psoriasis shampoos. I repeat: Wash your hair frequently; if not daily, at least four to six times per week.

COSMETICS

In general, I recommend use of as few cosmetics as possible. With regard to oily-skinned patients, especially those suffering from acne, I say cut them out altogether. If you absolutely must, stick to the water-base formulas offered by almost all companies these days. Mary Quant, Clinique, and Liquimat make good water-based products. Oil-based cosmetics are for dry skins or for older women whose complexions have developed the natural tolerance for oil that comes with age. Remember that all cosmetics are occlusive (pore clogging) to some degree. And clogged pores lead to acne (see Chapter 6).

A Regimen for Dry Skin

SOAPS

My advice for dry-skinned people is a regimen that avoids irritation and provides needed moisture while protecting what's already there. Wash only once a day. If you're really dry, dispense with soap altogether; use instead one of the excellent imitation soaps. Try Lowila Cake, Basis, and Oilatum. Alternately, you can stick with Dove, which is milder and less fatty and still doesn't cause drying. Be sure to avoid acne soaps that contain such drying agents as sulfur and tar. They'll defeat your purpose, as will deodorant soaps that contain halogenated salicylanilides and/or hexachlorophene. These latter substances work vigorously on the skin bacteria that cause sweat to smell. They also are quite irritating to dry skin.

ASTRINGENTS

Use none at all.

SHAMPOOS

Shampoo as infrequently as possible, since stripping oil and grease from the hair contributes to dry skin on the face. Dry-skinned people with particularly dry hair are sometimes happier with the nonalkaline (low detergent) shampoos that have been so widely advertised of late. This concept of low alkalinity is connected with the concept of the skin's pH level. The pH simply measures the acidity of the skin's surface; it's a scale from 1 (acid) to 14 (alkaline) and the normal face has a pH of 6.2. It is medically open to question whether or not the skin's pH is important or not. Traditionally, many dermatologists have felt that the skin has a normally acid pH (called the acid mantle) that should be protected against unduly alkaline substances. On the other hand, when alkalinity is reduced, the skin bacteria produce a surfeit of unionized fatty acids, which are highly irritating, especially for dry skin. So if your skin is dry, use one of the super fatted soaps mentioned above, such as Basis. Even "nonalkaline" shampoos are alkaline to some degree, so the fatted soaps are often better.

COSMETICS

The woman with dry skin has a higher tolerance for normally occlusive oil-based cosmetics. She can use more of them, and use them more frequently without running so high a risk of clogged pores and resulting pimples. I do not, however, recommend cosmetics as a cure for dry skin. Oily or dry, you're better off without them. Any moisturizer containing urea, an "aquaphilic" compound that both attracts water and prevents its loss, is the dry epidermis's best friend. Aquacare and Aquacare/HP (High Potency) are excellent.

A Regimen for Normal Skin

SOAPS

Well, you must be doing something right if your skin is normal! You can usually enjoy the benefits of deodorant soaps without worrying about drying or irritation. Washing twice a day with almost anything is good for you. Good soaps, from the standpoint of purity, are Ivory, Palmolive (regular, not Gold), and Aveeno Bar.

ASTRINGENTS

Only really necessary for oily skin, you can dispense with astringents, or at most use them once a day.

SHAMPOOS

As mentioned in the regimen for dry skin, a widely disputed concept once held that the skin and scalp had an "acid mantle" that somehow protected them. However, in my opinion the skin does not really have any such thing. Alkalinity was formerly thought to attack the skin's normal acid pH. Not so. The nonalkaline shampoos so touted of late are admittedly less detergent, but except for people with particularly dry or brittle hair, they provide protection you don't really need. The person with normal skin and hair can use anything off the drugstore shelf and rest easy that his or her hair isn't being ruined. Breck, Prell, VO-5, they're all perfectly fine.

COSMETICS

As it happens, most brands are formulated for "normal skin." But the cleanest, clearest-looking skin is that which breathes freely. You might have a higher tolerance for occlusive creams and makeups than an oily-skinned person, but I always recommend that my patients avoid cosmetics as a general rule.

All this attention to the epidermis is pointless if you neglect or unwittingly abuse the dermis that lies below. The dermis has its own set of vulnerabilities, which are generally the same whether the epidermis is oily or not.

The sun, for instance, can have very deleterious effects on the collagen and elastin contained in the dermis. These two proteins are the building blocks of dermal tissue and provide the dermal layers of the skin with the tone and resiliency that characterizes healthy skin. Sunlight in reasonable doses is good for the epidermis. In excessive doses over prolonged periods (often many years), it can cause premature aging, wrinkling, sagging, even scarring, by slowly destroying collagen and elastin. You can protect the dermis by judicious exposure to the sun and through the use of proper sunscreens. PreSun, Eclipse, and Uval are my favorites.

Diet directly affects the dermis, since the nourishment-carrying blood vessels are located in this level of the skin. Proper care of the dermis through diet means more than getting your vitamins and eating well-balanced meals. Vitamin C, incidentally, helps build collagen, one of the cornerstones of the dermis.

Some systemic medications can cause unforeseen damage. Systemic medications are those taken either orally or through injections, and they affect every organ in your system. This contrasts with topically (surface) applied medications whose effect is limited to the area of application. Cortisone is a notable example of a systemic medication taken by many people that has serious side effects on the dermal layers of the skin. It can cause purplish stretch marks, lead to poor healing, stimulate the oil glands (whose roots are in the dermis) to excessive oil production (an acnegenic condition), and weaken collagen proteins to boot! You should consult your physician on the effects of any systemic medication.

Hormones, particularly the estrogen in birth-control pills, can have bad side effects. Estrogen causes increased capillary growth and fragility. The capillaries are located in the dermis, and when too fragile, they can produce a bleeding into the skin and excess blood vessels called angiomas. Angiomas are the red spidery blotches on the face that afflict many women, especially during pregnancy. (Remember, birth-control pills actually simulate pregnancy within the body.)

Estrogen can also stimulate excess production of melanin, the protein that gives skin coloration. This can cause a brownish pigmentation on the face called chloasma, or the mask of pregnancy.

Alcohol leads to cherry angiomas too, at least indirectly. When consumed to excess, alcohol reduces the liver's ability to metabolize either the estrogens normally secreted by the woman's ovaries or the estrogenic hormones produced by the man's adrenals, resulting in the unsightly angiomas that blotch the face of many an alcoholic.

Tobacco takes its toll on the dermis too. Regular smokers suffer from a curious and imperfectly understood condition in which the collagen in the dermal tissue around the eyes is observed to be damaged. This results in crow's-feet.

Armed with a clearer picture of your skin and its susceptibilities, you're now ready for the inside information on some of the major factors influencing the condition of your skin.

Chapter 2

Hormones and Your Skin

The beauty of your skin is greatly influenced by hormones. These substances, whether produced by your own organ systems or introduced in pills or injections, critically affect both intracellular and extracellular fluid volume. This volume is reflected in what we call the "turgor" of the skin.

Skin with good turgor looks youthful and has a general tightness and firmness. Too much fluid leads to boggy, swollen-looking skin with enlarged pores. Too little fluid can result in the droopy, sagging skin associated with advancing age. Besides turgor, hormones also regulate such things as skin color, temperature, and cellular turnover rate. Certain deficiencies can result in skin that's cold and clammy, while excesses can make the skin hot and flushed.

The five hormones importantly associated with skin are androgens, estrogens, thyroid, steroids, and insulin. A description of each follows, along with a discussion of what they can do to and for your skin.

Androgens

The human body produces quite a selection of different androgens. These are male hormones produced in the testes, but women produce their own androgenic hormones in the adrenal gland. The androgenic hormone with greatest potency and effect is called testosterone.

Although androgens affect the whole skin, their influence is most noticeable on the face, pubic areas, and armpits. Too much androgen will make oil glands enlarge, thereby stimulating excess production of sebum. When that happens, the stage is set for acne, which results from clogged oil glands (see Chapter 6). As if acne were not enough, excess androgen also leads to hair loss on the head, while stimulating hair growth on the face.

Of course, to have these malfunctions, an actual surplus or deficiency of the hormone isn't really necessary. You may be entirely normal on the production end, but your oil glands or hair follicles may have an excessive response. This brings us again to the concept of "end organ sensitivity," which will reappear throughout the book. This concept revolves around the premise that every organ has a unique and not always predictable level of responsiveness. It explains why things like hair loss and acne are so selective. The same level of androgen in the bloodstreams of two people may well cause acne in one but not in the other. Why? Because the end organs involved (oil glands in the case of acne) have unique levels of susceptibility.

Although you want sufficient androgen levels for good turgor, excessive androgen is not desirable. There are a number of sources of androgen that lie outside the body.

Certain foods, like beef, liver, and wheat germ, may have high androgen content. Progesterone birth-control pills have the effect of high androgen, since the progesterone is metabolized into an androgen-like substance. Many women also receive injections of progesterone-like substances for other reasons. It's a common treatment for irregular menstrual periods and is used to initiate the regular cycle after childbirth. But in women, perhaps the most frequent source of excessive androgen—and the mysteriously sudden pimple—is stress. Stressful situations stimulate the adrenals, where androgenic hormones are produced. Result: an acnegenic condition in which the oil glands are overstimulated.

In relation to excessive androgen levels, I counsel avoidance of stress insofar as possible, avoidance of foods with high androgen content (see Chapter 6 for lists of acnegenic foods), and possibly a switch to estrogen-type birth-control pills. You should consult your doctor if you think your pills are giving you acne.

Estrogens

Estrogens are female hormones produced by the ovaries, and they have a variety of effects on the skin. Insofar as acne is concerned, estrogen-type birth-control pills are definitely superior to the progesterone type. The estrogen pills do seem to result in a tendency to gain weight, but they also reduce the sebum production of the oil glands, and at the same time enhance the turgor and elasticity of the skin. The result is a clear and moisturized complexion.

When a woman reaches age forty her body experiences a natural decline in estrogen production. That's when estrogen birth-control pills can be most effective. They do double duty, providing contraceptive protection while at the same time benefiting the skin. In fact, the administration of estrogen to menopausal women will often retard wrinkling and avert the dried-out appearance that characterizes aging skin. It also has a tranquilizing effect on older women and leads to a general feeling of well-being.

However, estrogen is not without its drawbacks. Although no experiments have conclusively associated it with cancer in humans, there have been experiments in which exogenously taken estrogens have caused cancers in laboratory animals. Medically prescribed systemic dosage of estrogen is known to retard certain hormone-responsive cancers (of the prostate and breast, for example) and is of use in treating heart disease. But estrogen treatments and/or pills are not recommended if you have clotting problems, high blood pressure, a history of stroke, or any existing cancer. Even if you're perfectly healthy, estrogen birth-control pills will photosensitize your skin, making it prone to chloasma. These are dark blotches that appear on the cheeks after sun exposure. They take months to go away, and sometimes are permanent!

When a woman is taking estrogen, any skin lesions she has—or might get—will be worse than if she were not taking estrogen. Moles get darker and bigger; papillomas (small benign skin tumors) can sprout up or become bigger if she has them already; blood vessels can appear on the surface of the skin, and sometimes burst into unsightly cherry angiomas.

However, for all this, there are many premenopausal women who are obviously estrogen deficient and will benefit greatly from estrogen treatment. How do you tell if you're one? Go to your doctor and have him test you by doing a smear of the cells of the uterus. If you're thin, have frail bones, irregular periods, small breasts, and narrow hips, there's a chance you're deficient. If you're heavy, big-boned, and have big hips, you've probably got plenty. Another way to tell is to have your doctor start you on an estrogen program and simply observe the results. If you see good effects, you most likely were deficient; if there are no observable effects, then you probably had plenty to start with and your problem requires a different solution. However, watch it; estrogens have side effects.

So far I've discussed only systemic estrogens, but the use of topical estrogen preparations deserves a word here. There is debate in medical circles as to whether it's really possible to deliver an effective dose of the hormone in this manner. The benefit would be the bypassing of many of the harmful side effects that take place when it's absorbed by the body. There are certain lotions, usually available by prescription, that purport to stop hair loss. They might work on some people, even though the estrogens they contain are considerably less potent than those in systemic medicines. Balding menopausal women probably have nothing to lose if they try an estrogen lotion for the scalp. But, in general, I advise you to avoid cosmetics that claim to deliver hormones to the skin. It is a dubious claim at best.

It is interesting to note the role of estrogen in premenstrual, menstrual, and/or postmenstrual flairs of acne. From the first day of the menstrual cycle, estrogen levels in a woman's body will steadily climb until mid-cycle. At that point, estrogen production begins to fall, while levels of progesterone begin to climb. The period begins as a response of the uterus to a lack of estrogen. And the probable reason for the acne flairs that so often occur during the period is a lack of estrogen to counteract the high accumulation of progesterone. Of course, every woman's curve varies, which is why acne flairs at different points for different women. Similarly, some women have a sufficiently high level of end organ sensitivity to avoid the acne flair altogether.

Thyroid

Now that amphetamines are regulated, thyroid has become a favorite prescription of diet doctors. The reason for this is the association of obesity with a lack of thyroid. But my feeling is that most people are fat because they eat too much, not because there's anything wrong with their glands.

Unbalanced levels of this hormone, produced by the gland of the same name, are very characteristic. If you have too much (hyperthyroid), the cutaneous blood flow will become greatly increased. This results in red, velvety feeling skin, and a persistent flushing of the face. Besides being hyperactive, you'll sweat a lot and possibly begin to note a thinning of the hair. In advanced cases of hyperthyroid, the skin can change color unpredictably (becoming either whiter or darker) and the nails can separate from the nail bed.

Hypothyroid, or the condition of too little thyroid, results in dry, brittle hair that tends to fall out, loss of eyebrows, and parchment-like, prematurely wrinkled skin. Both conditions respond well to treatment, and you can easily determine if thyroid imbalance is your problem by having your doctor administer T-3 and T-4 tests. These are tests for the presence of the hormone, but beware: If you're on the pill you must tell your doctor since it affects the outcome of the test.

Steroids

Your adrenal glands produce a wide variety of steroids, and people with too much or too little have skin that shows it only too well. Hypersteroid (when you have too much) can actually atrophy the skin. It becomes thin and shiny, gets lots of infections, is plagued with breaking blood vessels, and evidences poor healing. What's worse, steroids tend to stimulate the sebaceous oil glands, which increases the risk of acne. Hyposteroid (when you have too little) causes a loss of body hair, hyperpigmentation (darkening) of the skin, and sometimes a darkening of the nails as well.

A major cause of hypersteroid conditions is medication. Prednisone, which is literally a wonder drug in reducing inflammation and combatting allergic reactions, has many unpleasant side effects, namely edema (too much fluid in the skin), unduly ruddy and flushed complexion, the appearance of a buffalo hump on the back, and a coarsening of the facial features. People on Prednisone also fall prey to more yeast, fungal, and bacterial infections.

Many people take cortisone for allergic reactions and arthritis. It reduces the symptoms effectively, but cortisone also causes acne in from 80 percent to 90 percent of the people who take it. This is probably due to the fact that metabolized cortisone is highly androgenic. It is interesting to note here that stress-related acne is thought to derive in part from extra amounts of cortisone produced by the stress-activated adrenals.

Insulin

This hormone is produced by the pancreas, and a deficiency results in the common disease of diabetes. Insulin regulates the metabolism of carbohydrates, and if you can't metabolize them, your skin will manifest specific diabetic symptoms. These include a flushed complexion, persistent itching, necrobiosis lipoidica diabeticorum (yellow lesions described in Chapter 9), diabetic dermopathy (poor healing and brown lesions, also described in Chapter 9), and a tendency to break out in fungal, yeast, and bacterial infections, as well as boils!

Diabetes is easily regulated by insulin injections. The drawback to the injections is that they can lead to an atrophy of the skin and a depletion of subcutaneous fat layers in the areas of injection.

Chapter 3

How Diet Affects Your Skin

Many people believe that the skin can be fed externally by creams containing special oils, vitamins, and the like. This is not true. Healthy skin must be fed from inside by a bloodstream that contains proper nourishment. The condition of the skin can actually tell quite a bit about a person's diet. Acne can indicate a diet too heavy in hormones or iodides; a tendency to bruise often results from lack of vitamin C; dryness can sometimes be ascribed to vitamin A deficiency; and undue flushing or a red nose and cheeks are often the mark of too much alcohol consumption.

No miracle diet will give you good healthy skin. The best thing you can do for yourself is to eat a well-balanced diet without special supplements. To look good, skin only needs to be properly nourished. If it isn't, it heals poorly, bruises easily, looks dull and lifeless, is accompanied by brittle nails and bad hair. Ironically, many health-food diets contain the real junk to beware of, namely acnegenic (acne-causing) iodides and androgens.

The ideal diet for the skin is one that is light in iodine and heavy in essential polyunsaturated fatty acids. So I shall devote the balance of this chapter to describing these and other common elements of diet that help or hurt the skin.

Vitamin C

This vitamin, found abundantly in oranges and other citrus fruits, is one of the most essential to good skin. Its importance is illustrated by the story of why British sailors—and the nation at large by association—are called Limeys. It was the British who first discovered that scurvy, whose symptoms include bleeding gums and perifollicular hemorrhages (blood spots around the hair follicles), was caused by a lack of vitamin C. So sailors at sea were required to eat limes, and the Queen's navy went on to conquer the waters of the world. Vitamin C is crucial to the formation of collagen and elastin, both major proteins and building blocks of the dermis layer of the skin. Its absence leads to the leaky blood vessels that characterize scurvy, as well as poor wound healing in general.

Essential Fatty Acids

These are vitamins in all but name, and they insure the proper metabolism of the skin. Definitions first: The skin's metabolism is the process of building and shedding cells, at the right speed, in the right amounts. Fats are either saturated or polyunsaturated, depending on whether all links on the chemical carbon chain are attached to hydrogen molecules. If all are attached, the fat is called saturated; a good example is the fat on a piece of steak. It's pure cholesterol and leads directly to heart disease via obesity.

Polyunsaturated fats, however, are absolutely essential to healthy skin. Here, the carbon chains are missing hydrogen molecules, and the resulting substances are softer and more fluid. Cereal grains, nuts, margarine, and safflower or any other unsaturated oils are good examples. Whole milk is the best possible food for the skin since it's so rich in essential fatty acids. This fact was dramatized in a slightly incredible experiment in which babies were deprived of whole milk for the first twelve weeks of life. They were given skim milk instead, and the result was rapid development of dry, scaly skin. One is left wondering not so much about the effect of the milk, as whose babies they were. The experiment did however illustrate the importance of the high fatty acid content in milk and its correlation to good skin.

Oiliness of the skin is not affected by fat in the diet. It is a function of how sensitive the skin's oil glands are to hormone levels in the bloodstream. If you're to be a healthy animal, your diet must have enough fatty acids.

Zinc

This is a vital trace element that's ubiquitous in the average diet. It has been observed that zinc sulfate taken orally will help heal skin ulcers. Similarly, it's true that people with badly ulcerated skin usually have low levels of zinc in their systems. Therefore, although there are some questions about this, zinc is considered to increase the healing potential of the skin.

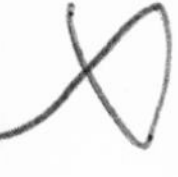

Vitamin K

Found in meat and green vegetables, vitamin K may sound obscure to you. However, it has a special importance to the skin, since it is required for the proper synthesis of the clotting factor in the bloodstream. Bruising is bleeding into the skin, and it's encouraged by a deficiency of vitamin K.

Vitamin A

We get our vitamin A from things like yellow vegetables (carrots, squash), and fish (mostly cod) liver oil. It acts as an invaluable aid to skin metabolism, which when defective can cause such conditions as psoriasis or even skin cancer in animals. Vitamin A deficiencies are actually rather common, particularly one called toadskin. Sufferers of this have goosebump-like accentuations of the hair follicles. Lack of vitamin A can also thicken the skin, sometimes blocking off oil and sweat glands.

Alternately, it's possible to take an excess of vitamin A (and a pigment called carotene) into the system. This can cause a yellowing of the horny layer of the skin, particularly around the eyes and on the palms, that's often taken for jaundice. In true jaundice, however, the whites of the eyes become yellow. Not so with an excess of vitamin A. Of course, some people's systems just can't metabolize a normal intake of vitamin A, which results in a yellowing of the skin. In my practice, I see this about once every other month.

Retinoic acid (which is vitamin A) is incidentally the current rage for treating acne. Applied topically (to the skin's surface) it tends to keratinize (harden) the oil glands and hinder oil production while turning existing pimples into unsightly slushy pustules. This usually brings about a marked eventual improvement in the acne, but only after an initial period during which the skin is not pretty.

Iron

This important nutrient is found in green vegetables and red meats. Liver would be an especially good source if it didn't contain so much cholesterol and androgen. A deficiency of iron can lead to hair loss and uncomfortably dry skin. If extreme, it can bring on what's called Plummer-Vinson syndrome, which is marked by a difficulty in swallowing, hair loss, and fingernails that become spooned (concave).

Protein

Without the protein building blocks called amino acids, skin will tend to stretch and droop, won't heal well, and will wrinkle early. Hair tends to fall out too. The intensity of these symptoms depends on the degree of protein deprivation. Proteins are found in both meat and vegetable inputs of a balanced diet. Milk, mentioned earlier as the best food for the skin, is rich not only in essential fatty acids, but also in zinc and protein.

It should be clear by now that an improper diet can damage the skin. This damage can be worse than you think. Watch out for the following:

Beware of Foods with High Androgen Content

Androgens are sex-related hormones produced by women and men that cause pimples. The cause is indirect, since androgens actually stimulate the skin's oil glands to excessive oil secretion. This in turn heightens the probability of plugged-up oil glands, which then become pimples.

The androgens you produce play a necessary role in your own body that outweighs their effect on the oil glands. However, many commercially grown foodstuffs are fed steroids and estrogens that, chemically, are nearly identical to androgens. These can cause a similar overstimulation of the oil glands, as can the androgen content of many birth-control pills. Your body's tolerance for these substances can be easily exceeded by diets with either artificially introduced androgens or by foods that are naturally androgenic, such as wheat germ, shellfish, organ meats such as liver and kidney, and sweetbreads. Pork and lamb should be popular meats for the skin. Likewise, most fish (*not* shellfish) are equally androgen-free.

Beware of Vitamin E

Vitamin E is a fad favorite these days, and I myself have been convinced by cardiologist friends that it does prevent heart attacks. At least it can't hurt when taken internally. But I feel that it can do damage when applied topically. It has not been proven to promote healing. The only experiments along these lines have been done with rats, and they are not conclusive.

However, vitamin E is known to be highly allergenic. This was dramatically illustrated not too long ago when a major toiletries company introduced a vitamin E deodorant. This product caused such widespread sensitization to vitamin E that it had to be removed from circulation. Systemic vitamin E has upon occasion helped in rare skin diseases, for instance the yellow-nail syndrome, which I doubt you'll ever encounter. Otherwise, its main virtue is as an instant sales promoter among the unwary. I say don't put it on your skin; it doesn't work.

Beware of Blushing Foods

This category includes anything that's hot and spicy—chili, curry, hot peppers—as well as the caffeine in tea and coffee and the alcohol in wine and liquor. These elements all have one thing in common: They cause vasodilatation, or the expansion of the blood vessels. Now I'm not recommending that you eliminate any of these things from your diet. I am telling you that a prolonged diet of blushing foods can cause the blood vessels to remain permanently expanded. Then you've got a condition called acne rosacea—a big red nose—and visible swollen capillaries close to the skin surface. And if you've already got this kind of trouble from some other cause, then blushing foods will only make it worse.

Beware of Dangerously Low Calorie Levels

Subcutaneous fat is very important to the appearance of your skin. Without it, the skin appears withered, dry, rough, inelastic, cold, and dead to the touch. Although these signs are associated with old age, they can be observed in younger people who are calorie deprived.

The disease called kwashiorkor, whose rashes and dryness give the skin a crazy-pavement look, is essentially starvation. Kwashiorkor would seem to be limited to parts of the world with acute poverty and food shortages. However, another disease, anorexia nervosa, whose symptoms resemble those of starvation, is suffered by countless women of affluence who compulsively diet. The skin of these women also tends to be dry, rough, scaly, and inelastic.

An experimental diet of 1570 calories daily for twenty-three weeks resulted in poor skin with the characteristics mentioned above, plus hair that became dull and dry and had a tendency to stop growing and fall out. Vitamin supplements, even massive ones, will not avert this apparent premature aging of the skin and hair. In young people, the damage is reversible with weight gain, but it becomes less so with age. So beware the slick line in the women's magazines that knowingly advises you to stay fifteen pounds less than the doctor's schedule of "normal weights." Do so if you want to, but be prepared for the price your skin must inevitably pay for long periods of continuous underweight.

Beware of Artificial Sweeteners

In and of themselves, sugar substitutes won't hurt you, and under the right circumstances they are excellent aids to weight loss. However, they are photosensitizers. This means that certain susceptible individuals can get a helluva sunburn by drinking diet sodas in the sun. Not only is there an increased predisposition toward sunburn, but burns of this sort often leave behind blotchy dark marks called hyperpigmentation, which can be permanent. Although we all have different susceptibilities and tolerance levels, and some of us won't notice this effect, enough do suffer to make this warning an important one.

Beware of Phytophoto Dermatitis

This warning applies to those elements of your diet that you spill on yourself! Some plants have oils that are highly photosensitizing when applied to the skin externally. Lime juice causes about the most dramatic burn, but figs, parsnip, fennel, dill, parsley, and carrots will do about the same. Again, these are foods that require external application to the skin under sunlight in order for adverse effects to be noted.

Beware of Obesity

Too much fat makes an individual prone to eczema, rashes, and fungal infections. The reason for this is that fat people sweat too much. This generally fouls up the body's own systems of self-disinfection and renders the fat person an easy target for skin irritation and infection.

Beware of Vitamin Deficiencies

Some mention has already been made of vitamin deficiencies, but a number of common complaints stem from a specific lack of the B-complex vitamins.

A sufficient lack of niacin, contained in whole grain products, causes the three Ds: dermatitis, diarrhea, and dementia (madness). Pellagra, a disease characterized by rashes on the face and the tops of the hands, stems from deprivation of niacin.

A lack of riboflavin, which is contained in dairy products and red meats, results in what's called the oro-oculo-genital syndrome. This is characterized by a whitening of the pigmentation around the corners of the mouth, redness and a moist, greasy feel to the skin on the top of the cheeks, and lesions in the scrotum.

Insufficient vitamin B_6 results in seborrhea—lesions, scaling, and greasiness around the nose. We normally get needed vitamin B_6 from milk, meat, and the whole grains in bread, bran, and flour products.

Finally, a lack of vitamin B_{12} leads to hypopigmentation (lightening of the skin) in the extremities and pernicious anemia. Important sources of B_{12} vitamins are red meats, especially liver.

Beware of Alcohol

Immoderate and prolonged use of alcohol will first ruin the liver, and when that's accomplished, the skin will be rendered defenseless as follows. The liver metabolizes numerous substances that would otherwise cause skin damage. Estrogen and estrogen-like substances produced in both sexes provide a vivid example. If your liver is ruined through a life of heavy drinking, high levels of unmetabolized estrogen will occur in your system. Estrogen causes vasodilatation, or expansion and increased permeability of the blood vessels. This leads to spiders, those unsightly burst capillaries just below the skin surface. High estrogen levels also result in gynecomastia, the medical term for breast enlargement in males, as well as acne rosacea, the large red nose mentioned earlier.

That's not all. A liver debilitated by alcohol is similarly unable to metabolize androgen and androgen-like substances. This can lead to hair loss, since excess androgen will tend to involute the hair follicles. Yellow jaundice is yet another condition of the skin related to a damaged liver. It's caused by unmetabolized bile products in the system. These bile products can also lead to uncomfortable itching.

Beware of High Cholesterol

Immoderate consumption of high cholesterol foods (milk, butter, beef) can cause little fatty tumors on the skin called xanthomas. These are colored from yellow to red to white and come in five different varieties, each corresponding to a specific elevation of blood fat level.

Xanthelasma, for instance, is a condition of little white to yellow papules on the eyelids. They're nothing but fat, and more than half of the people who demonstrate this symptom have too much cholesterol in the blood. At its worst, a cholesterol level this high can kill you through heart disease, in which similar fatty tumors will form in the blood vessels.

But xanthomas can appear anywhere—on tendons, hands, and bony prominences—and if you see them, go directly to your doctor for a lipid (fat) profile of the blood. This is particularly important for men, who are most likely to be victims of fatal heart attacks. For reasons not fully understood, the natural estrogen levels in women seem to protect them from similarly induced attacks. You'll almost never hear of a premenopausal woman having a heart attack.

A Special Weight-Loss Diet That's Kind to Your Skin

A proper weight level is important, but so is a balanced diet. You don't want to deprive your skin of needed vitamins and nutrients, but neither do you want a diet heavy in androgenic health foods, super vitamin supplements with too many acnegenic iodides or photosensitizing artificial sweeteners. For a low calorie weight-loss diet that won't hurt the skin, try the following:

Breakfast. Half a grapefruit or a small glass of juice (for vitamin C); half a bowl of Special K (for calories and vitamins); an egg once or twice a week; coffee with whole milk (for fatty acids) and a spoonful of sugar (which won't kill you once in a while!).

Lunch. Cottage cheese (for fatty acids, minerals, and protein) with fruit or a green vegetable; or alternate this with any plain fish dish (*not* shellfish). Beverage: water only.

Afternoon snack. Skip the caffeine or saccharin that you can't escape in coffee or diet soda; have a piece of fresh fruit instead.

Dinner. Salad with lemon juice (for vitamin C); a meat dish, preferably veal (second choice is chicken, third is beef, but don't buy prime; stick to the low-fat cuts labeled choice or good); a small baked potato with margarine; a French cruller or two cookies for dessert; alternate each day between a glass of whole milk and one of skim.

Chapter 4

Stress: Your Skin's Worst Enemy

Stress born of the cares of daily living can truly wreak havoc with the skin. Our emotions aren't just pinned on our collective sleeves; they're literally branded on the flesh! This is only logical, since skin is the physical interface between ourselves and our environment. It not only mirrors human adjustment to the physical circumstances of life, but it's also a window into the individual's inner condition. Many people who come to the doctor seeking explanations of rashes, eruptions, or hives actually are often suffering from nothing more than stress, tension, and psychological unhappiness.

Your system is replete with nerve endings. In the skin there are specific receptors for touch, pressure, heat, and pain, and the appropriate nerve endings are distributed logically. For example, you have considerably more touch-sensitive fibers in your fingertips than in your rear end. Nevertheless, stimulation of a strong enough nature can provoke the same reaction from nerves not designed to perceive that particular stimulus. Get hit hard enough and your heat sensors will register pain; get scorched badly enough and your pressure sensors will register heat. And get nervous enough and all the sensors will react to the stress.

Now, particularly in the case of stress, the skin is capable of demonstrating a bewildering array of reactions. And if I call these reactions psychosomatic, I don't mean to suggest that they aren't real. The pain and embarrassment are certainly real. So real, in fact, that most patients of common stress-induced conditions refuse to believe that their symptoms are being cooked up in their own heads. They insist they are suffering from, or are allergic to, something. Tell me what it is, they say.

The following discussion of the most common stress-related diseases is arranged in order from the most psychologically induced to the least psychologically induced. Many readers, I am sure, will think this a collection of obscure lunatic reactions—at least until they come to a condition that has always troubled them! I repeat, these are all exceedingly common complaints, which I treat daily.

Trichotilomania. This condition typically (though not exclusively) afflicts young women and children. Often a concerned mother will bring the patient in and say, "Doctor, my daughter is losing her hair." I look at the girl, and her hair seems quite normal and healthy, except for a small, well demarcated patch, usually on the side of the scalp. On that patch, sure enough, she seems to be balding. Many sufferers will even bring in a little fuzzy ball of hair!

Why is this healthy young girl losing her hair? Because she's pulling it out herself, that's why! This explanation is regularly rejected by the patient as too absurd. In point of fact, she may be unconsciously twirling a doomed strand with her fingertips at the same time she's talking to me. So what can I recommend? A tranquilizer. Sometimes, a doctor will suture a bandage over the affected area to prove to the patient that her hair will grow beneath the bandage when it's protected from unconscious yanking. This is a radical procedure that I do not recommend. Aside from the fact that more than half the patients so treated will undoubtedly find some excuse for picking the bandage off, those that don't might be driven to some unexpected excess when deprived of the symptom. Even though the patient will often seem entirely normal, the trichotilomania is an important outlet for some suppressed stress or conflict. What's clearly needed is something—be it drugs or therapy or whatever—to calm this person down.

Before I leave the subject, let me note that the condition can apply to hair anywhere on the body. I see people almost as frequently who claim to be losing their pubic hair!

Delusions of Parasitosis. Stress is clearly written all over the faces of these sufferers. They think the world is against them and make no pretense otherwise. Like the trichotilomanic girls with the balls of hair, they come with bags or little boxes filled with bits of hair and unidentifiable crusty fragments. They complain that their skin is infested with worms, bugs, and similar parasites.

The first thing I do is take a blood test. Even though this condition is almost always delusions of parasitosis, occasionally it is actually caused by a nutritional problem. I ask questions about the patient's diet and sometimes get the wildest answers. Some people subsist on gin and sandwiches, it seems. Diets like this can cause vitamin deficiencies, like pellagra (lack of niacin), whose symptoms are dermatitis and diarrhea.

Too frequently the patient manifests the same symptoms as pellagra, but does not have it. The blood test is OK, and it remains for me to convince an increasingly suspicious patient that there is nothing physically wrong with him or her despite the seeming dryness of the skin and the box of "evidence." Once again, these are people who need to be calmed down, by tranquilizers or other methods. Delusions of parasitosis, incidentally, is three times as frequent in my practice as trichotilomania.

Syphilophobia. I see this almost every day too, and it's a similar situation to those already cited. Remember that these are conditions that people deem serious enough to bring to a dermatologist! Briefly, syphilophobia is the conviction that some spot, which can be located anywhere on the body, is syphilitic. The visit to my office always follows some situation that has caused extreme guilt. For instance, the young boy who has just lost his virginity or the married man who has just had his first affair. Sometimes a man who has had a benign spot on his thigh for the last thirty years will be unfaithful for the first time and presto, the spot begins to itch. He says "Oh, my God" and calls for an appointment. Perhaps city doctors see more of this than doctors in the less anonymous suburbs, where families and friends might somehow hear of the visit.

Lichen Chronicus Simplex. The medical profession loves to label "simplex" those conditions whose causes lie totally beyond anyone's understanding. Not-so-simplex would be more appropriate. This condition of chronic rashes around the neck, elbows, and frequently on the legs below the kneecap is one of the most common complaints in dermatology.

Here we have a situation where the doctor looks for a

cause and just can't find anything. It ably demonstrates the "itch-scratch-itch" syndrome. The skin itches so you scratch it; then the scratch seems to make it itch more. But why? Well, there is no physical reason. But there is a common reaction to stress that we all demonstrate at some time or another. We fold our arms and nervously handle our own elbows. And by extension, when we lie in bed at night we will nervously rub our lower legs first with one foot, then the other, while we wrangle with our problems. How does skin that's been rubbed react? It becomes thicker. Gradually, unconsciously, the rubbed skin becomes lichenized, or horny. Lichenification means accentuation of skin markings, which is where this condition gets its name. My own prescription is relaxation and application of antipruritic topical medications.

Acne Excorié des jeunes filles. The name is in French since the condition was first described there. It is commonly noted in high-strung adolescent girls and consists of unsightly acne and pockmarks. The regular dose of adolescent acne is made worse when stress enters the picture. It's believed that stress stimulates the adrenals, resulting in increased production of steroids. This causes increased oil production by the skin's sebaceous oil glands. The excess oil arrives on skin that's usually already too oily, and it leads to more occluded (clogged) pores and pimples.

Some young girls are under such stress from life that they actually gouge out (excoriate) the pimples with their fingernails. Sounds terrible, doesn't it? And we doctors see it every week.

The Sweat Retention Syndrome. This would be more properly labeled the sweat tension syndrome. Sweating is intimately related to the nervous system. Cut certain nerves to any area of the body, and that area will not sweat. By observing where a patient does and does not sweat, a doctor can often locate a tumor on the spinal cord.

Stress will usually cause perspiration in the following favorite areas: armpits, anogenital area, palms, and soles. Before I go further, you should also understand that sweat is essentially weak urine. It's 99 percent water, plus urea, and small amounts of sodium, chloride, potassium, and lactate. Symptoms of the syndrome are evidenced, for example, by the patient with hand eczema. This is a red, scaly rash along the sides of the fingers, accompanied by what appears to be water bubbles. The sufferer says it only happens when he or she is nervous. Sometimes it attacks the feet as well and is assumed to be athlete's foot.

You've probably guessed by now that the bubbles aren't full of water; they're full of sweat. These people are producing so much sweat that it literally all can't get out the pore openings. Like a traffic jam at rush hour, the secretion of sweat is occurring at such a rate that the normal gland openings clog up, forcing the sweat to collect in irritating bubbles below the surface. Sometimes it will only happen on a single finger. Interestingly, I frequently see patients with this symptom under the wedding ring! Other times, the blocked perspiration gathers into a huge blister on the hand that goes by the name of pompholyx.

People who perspire excessively impair their own mechanisms for self-disinfecting. Skin that is dry and healthy is also bacteriostatic, which means that it does not encourage multiplication of bacteria. Sweaty people have a tendency to have many more bacterial and fungus reactions, things like crotch rot.

I can suggest several things for hyperhidrosis. While there are prescription anti-inflammatory creams that do help, the patient needs most of all to calm down, and I emphasize that fact as strongly as possible. Pills are available to reduce sweating. Unfortunately, they also increase temperature and interfere with the central nervous system, so I'm not fond of them. Sometimes, a person will sweat so much that sympathetic nerve fibers alongside the spinal cord must be surgically severed. This is rare, though. Most treatments consist of tranquilizers, creams, and a topically applied 25 percent aluminum chloride tincture. The tincture can be prepared at your drugstore, contains the same ingredient that stops wetness in nationally advertised deodorants (aluminum chloride), and is, all in all, an excellent inexpensive deodorant.

Bruises. "I get black and blue marks when I'm nervous," and "I had a terrible fight with my boyfriend and got this tremendous bruise, but I don't know how," are two basic themes heard every week. Stress often leads to increased capillary fragility. Bruises are simply bleeding into the skin. They are considerably more likely to occur if the capillary system's normal permeability is increased, which is what happens when you're nervous. Along with the capillary fragility, stress also leads to vasodilatation, or dilation of the blood vessels. The increase of blood flow caused by the enlarged vessels not only exacerbates the more fragile capillary walls, but also plays an important part in the following condition.

Hives. People who get unexpected bruises after emotional fights will sometimes get hives too. Hives, sweat, eczema, and bruises are the unhappy lot of a too-stressful life, and vasodilatation plays a pivotal part.

The increased amount of blood in the skin, which results from the dilation of the blood vessels, tends to make it more likely that you will react to some external stimulant or allergen. The dust or cat hair or what-have-you that might have no effect under normal circumstances seems to have a higher likelihood of causing irritation with the increased exposure to the bloodstream that results from vasodilatation.

Urticaria (hives) are reddish welts on the skin usually surrounded by a paler area. They are the classic example of what's called the wheal and flare response. This reaction is normal in a healthy person. The wheal is a bump that arises from a scratch or abrasion. The initial bump will then flair, or spread out. This response is mediated by the nerve network in the skin, and like the capacity to perspire, it ceases when the nerves serving the area are cut.

The most common of skin diseases, hives most commonly afflicts women. Although both sexes suffer, women between thirty-five and forty-five years of age have the worst time with hives. The wheal and flare of hives is a reaction to something, but the problem is rather more subtle than it seems at first. Most doctors put their patients on elimination diets on the assumption that a case of hives is purely an allergic reaction. In my opinion, 80 percent of the time it's a case of nerves and stress that no diet's going to help.

Hives can, of course, be allergically related—about 15 percent to 20 percent of the time, it's an obvious reaction to a new drug or a can of cherry soda. And there are also cases in which the uncomfortable welts are manifestations of exotic diseases. But, I repeat, 80 percent of the time, a bout with hives is caused by stress, unhappiness, and anxiety. I usually discover that along with the hives the patient also thinks his or her life is a waste, his or her job is terrible, and his or her spouse hates him or her.

The best treatment for hives is one that calms the

patient down. Often there is nothing to do but prescribe mild tranquilizers, such as Valium or Librium. Unfortunately, about nine out of ten people who visit my office are already taking Valium or Librium, which means I must upgrade the assault and prescribe an even stronger tranquilizer. Some people are so anxiety-ridden that they need two or three major tranquilizers a day. This is not good, but under certain circumstances it is better than hives.

Of course, most hive cases are not so dramatic. The cells in the skin called mast cells contain tiny granules of histamine. This substance causes leaky blood vessels and contributes to the edema (excess fluid collection) that is characteristic of hive-afflicted skin. Therefore, when normal wheal and flare reaction occurs under stressful circumstances (and resulting vasodilatation), it will very likely turn into a hive. And if you suffer from hives, don't take aspirin. Aspirin may make hives worse.

Shingles. Herpes zooster (pronounced zoster) is the medical name for the painful groups of red blisters called shingles. The disease is caused by a virus, and chances are you're walking around with the virus right now!

It is the same virus that causes chicken pox, but if you never had chicken pox, you'll never suffer from shingles. What happens after childhood chicken pox is a suppression of the virus by antibodies developed in your bloodstream. However, this is only suppression, not eradication. These viruses burrow away into nerve roots near the spinal cord and can remain there unnoticed for years.

This disease is a model example of the interaction between skin and nerves. Not only does the virus inhabit the nerve tissues, but nervous stress worsens the condition and often causes it in the first place. In extreme cases, when the body's normal antibody defenses are breached by medication or cancer, the shingles become generalized and spread all over the body. Usually, however, shingles are limited and localized, often brought on by a physical, mental, or traumatic shock (like a car crash) or a stressful situation.

The condition has two phases. At first, during a period of from one to three weeks, a victim notes the redness and blisters. Both young and old are afflicted, but older people usually have more pain. The second phase, however, almost exclusively attacks older people. It's called post shingles pain, occurs about six months after the initial outbreak, and can be absolutely excruciating.

Usually I won't give a sixty-five-year-old patient pain-killing steroids because of the side effects. But sometimes the risk is not as great as the potential of post shingles pain. Interestingly, there's a way to determine how bad the pain is going to be months before it comes. One can inject a small amount of histamine into the skin and watch for the familiar wheal and flare response. The wheal will usually be noted promptly. But if severe pain is going to come in the months ahead, the flare reaction will not occur. Then I'll usually prescribe steroids.

Hair Loss. Stress causes hair loss. It's as simple as that. The normal head will shed 100 to 200 hairs each day, while the stressful head will lose 500. Why the hair follicle does this is a mystery, especially since the follicle itself never dies. It always maintains the potential to grow new hair.

Stress does more than just accelerate normal hair loss. You've heard of the person so traumatized that his hair turned white overnight? Well, this is approximately true. Shock can actually cause the hair to fall completely out. The new hair that grows back is white or gray. Stress can also exacerbate an exotic allergic reaction called alopecia areata. Alopecia sufferers have developed a temporary allergy to their own hair. This is quite common, accounting for bald patches the size of a half-dollar on the scalps of many young women between twenty and thirty. It very frequently occurs after a death in the family.

Lichen Planus. At this end of the list, I'm getting into diseases that are related to stress without necessarily being exclusively caused by it. Lichen planus, which is a condition of violet and reddish papules commonly located on the wrists, ankles, and other extremities, has confusing causes. Sometimes certain medications will bring it on, but usually almost all sufferers have had a recent death in the family, have lost their job, or are laboring under some similarly stressful burden.

Lichen planus is ugly and can last for months. Even when it finally goes away, it is apt to leave marks of hyperpigmentation (darkening) behind. "Calm down" is, of course, the most valid advice I can offer in this case. Fortunately, however, I can also prescribe topical steroids, which actually do help the condition somewhat. Steroids cause vasoconstriction and less itching.

Vitiligo. Melanocytes are cells that produce melanin, which causes pigmentation of the skin. Vitiligo is a disease in which the patient apparently becomes allergic to his own melanocytes. The symptoms are a sudden loss of color in patches on the skin. It's most obvious in black-skinned people, but lighter complexioned people get it too.

Vitiligo can often be a physical response to a mental trauma of some sort. Your system, for reasons unknown, will develop antibodies that fight your own melanin-producing melanocytes. There is nothing really to be done about it either. Many doctors prescribe topical steroids, which usually don't do much. Others quite honestly attempt no medication and simply wait for the pigment to return idiopathically (which translates as "mysteriously").

Stress Pimples. Pimples are caused by clogged oil glands. Stress stimulates production of steroids within your body, and these steroids can stimulate the production of oil in the sebaceous glands of the face. The stress pimple is really no different from a normal pimple, but it arises in circumstances (i.e., excessive oiliness) that are due chiefly to stress. Especially on the night of the Big Date, when you use extra pore-clogging makeup, the hyperoiliness brought on by stress can make a pimple almost inevitable.

Chapter 5

Cosmetics: The Pros and Cons

Even as a dermatologist, I'm sometimes confused by all the night creams, day creams, foundations, clarifying lotions, brush-ons and blush-ons. The language that describes these products is usually pure mumbo jumbo and throws very little light on the ultimate effect they'll have on your skin. So for understanding's sake, I'll first divide *familia cosmetica* into the four following categories.

Creams. To illustrate immediately a confusing cosmetic description, please note that what's called a hydrophilic ointment happens to be a cream! Creams can be described as oil-in-water mixtures. They are usually white; they tend to vanish; they are greaseless. Hydrophilic ointment, for example, contains a substance that attracts available moisture. This is very different from moisturizers that coat the skin, plug the pores, and hold moisture in. Creams by themselves do not moisturize well; when rubbed on rough hands they will make the skin feel better temporarily, then promptly and completely vanish.

Lotions. Lotions are also oil-in-water preparations. They are neither greaseless nor occlusive (pore-clogging).

Ointments. Water-in-oil preparations are called ointments. They are greasy and occlusive. The most effective moisturizers are ointments and they're good for dry skin.

Powders. They are occlusive, and as you know, this can cause acne.

At best, cosmetics are successful aids to beauty and grooming. Used tastefully, they can certainly make you look beautiful. However, they can—and usually do—mess up your complexion.

Before anyone becomes frightened, I hasten to state that cosmetics really present no danger to the organism. All manufacturers go to painstaking lengths to assure that their products are hypoallergenic. Whether the product is marketed as hypoallergenic or not, you can be sure that the manufacturer conducted extensive tests to determine the incidence of allergic reaction to every ingredient in each formula he sells. No one wants to be sued.

I was once a candidate myself in a manufacturer's "maximum sensitization test." Any company with a new product will immediately set out to test it on a sample of virgin volunteers. The product is first broken down into its individual ingredients. Next, the volunteers (who have never been in a test) have a solution of sodium lauryl sulfate applied to the skin. This irritating solution removes the top two or three layers of the epidermis, thereby enhancing the possibility of allergic reaction. Each separate ingredient is applied to an individual volunteer in high intensities under occlusion. This means that they spread on much more than you'd ever apply yourself, then seal the site with strong tape. These tests are repeated several times on each volunteer and the results are watched as closely as possible. Every ingredient in the product is assigned a sensitizing index, which translates as the number of people who have an allergic reaction (become sensitized) per thousand attempts at sensitization. Even under the maximized sodium lauryl tests, the average sensitizing index for a typical cosmetic ingredient is between .01 and .03. Or, one to three people have allergic reactions per 100,000 users of the product.

All cosmetic makers engage in these extensive tests (required incidentally by the Federal Drug Administration) whether they label their products hypoallergenic or not. It is sometimes true that costly hypoallergenic formulas have fewer allergenic ingredients. On the other hand, an "allergenic" ingredient in a regular non-hypoallergenic product has such a low sensitizing index as to be statistically quite safe. The big myth of expensive hypoallergenic cosmetics deserves to be shot down. Unless you are an extraordinarily allergic person, they certainly do not justify the extra cost. Almost every company does the same tests, and they all keep complaint files so as to quickly remove from circulation any product that demonstrates undue allergenic incidence. What's more, the exotic hypoallergenic products marketed by many smaller companies are actually manufactured (and tested) by the big companies, which have huge manufacturing capabilities and will make up any formula presented to them.

Allergic Reactions

Despite all the testing, allergic reactions are a major drawback to using cosmetics. First of all, there are two types of allergic reactions: immediate and delayed. Immediate reactions are like the hives that erupt right after you eat strawberry ice cream or anything else to which you might be allergic. Antibodies borne by the blood cause the reaction as soon as the allergenic substance enters the bloodstream. A substance called phenolphthalein causes many eruptions of this sort. You may think you've never touched the stuff, but if you've ever taken a laxative or indulged in cheap red wine (colored with it), you have!

Delayed allergic reactions, logically enough, take more time to manifest themselves. Poison ivy, for example, will wait a day before it starts to blister. But before you have any sort of allergic reaction, you must first be *sensitized.* The allergic reaction itself is caused by antibodies produced in your system to combat substances the system perceives as foreign. Sometimes sensitization occurs as a result of first exposure. So, the second exposure is marked by the allergic reaction. Sometimes the allergic response doesn't show up until the fourth exposure, or the fortieth, or the four hundreth. The skin is eccentric and people don't always sensitize at the same rate.

I have many older patients who come to my office and say, "Doctor, I've been using this product for thirty years and all of a sudden it's giving me a rash!" This illustrates an interesting part of cosmetic making. Manufacturers, well aware that continued application of anything will eventually result in sensitization, are constantly altering the formulas of their products. You might not be able to tell the difference, but every six to eighteen months the ingredients of most cosmetics, including your favorites, are very slightly altered. Inevitably, there will be isolated reactions among some users who are allergic to whatever new was added!

The ability to have allergies, strange as it may seem at

first, is crucial to the organism's ability to live. The body is constantly producing little cancers, stray little cells, that are fortunately perceived as dangerous. They are destroyed by antibodies in what is essentially an allergic response. When the body's ability to single out and destroy these dangerous cells declines, as it does with age, you get cancer.

Allergic reactions are sometimes baffling and their causes quite unexpected. It seems logical to assume that the major cause of scaly red dermatitis around the eyes is irritating mascara, right? Wrong. The main cause of this type of dermatitis is nail polish. Don't try to flick something off your eyelash when your nails are wet. Some people suffer from rashes in the groin and armpits, a condition that is often the result of irritating ingredients in certain soaps. Sometimes soap just doesn't get completely washed off in those areas. Often an allergic reaction is not even caused by a major ingredient. It may be the emulsifying agent, the preservatives, the perfume, or the vehicle base. There are so many ingredients in the average cosmetic that your reaction to one may be confusingly masked by your reaction to another! And you may unwittingly sensitize yourself to obscure ingredients.

An interesting and unusual case occurred last year in New York City. The case was a minor epidemic of poison ivy on the feet! Poison ivy demonstrates the classical allergic reaction. The first time you touch it, there's never a problem. You could bathe a baby in it! The second time, watch out. The allergenic substance in poison ivy (*Rhus toxicodendron*), called rhus, is also found in the skin of mangoes. There is, in fact, a mango dermatitis, which consists of blisters around the mouths of careless mango eaters. The New York occurrence witnessed scores of girls from Queens afflicted with terrible cases of poison ivy on the soles of their feet. The mystery was solved when a common factor was noted about each girl. They had all recently bought leather sandals at a Greenwich Village boutique. The sandals were imported from India where they had been tanned with ingredients containing rhus!

Young pharmacology students are constantly searching for a wonder product to make them rich. The strange history of vitamin E deodorant is an interesting example of what can happen. Sweat is quite odorless, at least until the skin bacteria begin to work on it. Vitamin E is an antioxidant, and some bright researcher quite logically supposed that application of an antioxidant would stop bacterial oxidation. It did, but the product also resulted in massive sensitization to vitamin E, with attendant allergic symptoms.

Mechanical depilatories (hair removers) are very popular these days. Doubtless you've heard of (or been) one of the many people who have tried "waxing." This process to remove unwanted hair consists of painting on hot wax, then pulling it off when dry. If the petrochemicals in the wax don't get you, there's a good chance the perfumes, resins, or adhesives will. Result: allergic reaction, commonly manifested as small red bumps around the hair follicles.

Another very common allergenic substance is paraphenylenediamine, or PPDA. It's found in permanent oxidation-type hair dyes. Many states require beauticians to give a patch test for PPDA before coloring your hair. Other common causes of allergic reactions are nail polish lacquers, perfumes, and lipsticks.

Primary Irritant Dermatitis

A primary irritant is a substance that irritates the skin's surface. For example, turpentine applied to your arm will cause a rash. It is highly irritating. This rash is not to be confused with an allergic reaction. You must first be sensitized to a substance before your body will produce antibodies that combat that substance allergically. The resulting allergic reaction is caused by the antibodies in the bloodstream, not by irritation of the skin's surface. Unfortunately, a good many cosmetics, even when they don't cause allergic reactions, do contain irritating ingredients. The resulting dermatitis constitutes another good reason not to use them.

Perspiration odor, a major target of the cosmetic industry, provides an interesting example of the widespread use of a primary irritant. Aluminum chloride is the active ingredient in many antiperspirant and deodorant products. This is tough stuff, as a lot of people with sore armpits will testify! The latest thinking on sweat glands has it that the perspiration is drawn out of the gland by electromagnetic forces. Each of your sweat glands, incidentally, is between six and eight inches long. The proximal end, buried within the bottom layers of the dermis, is thought to have a positive electrical charge. The distal end, or the surface opening, is negatively charged. Each gland is incredibly coiled and surrounded by blood vessels. Water from the blood moves through cellular walls and into the gland by osmosis. It's the opposing polarity of each end of the sweat gland that is thought to somehow move the perspiration out onto the skin's surface.

Aluminum chloride, in fact all the aluminum salts, change the polarity of the sweat gland. Without the negative charge, the magnetic attraction is eliminated. And presto! Perspiration simply stops coming to the surface. Whatever else this does to you, it really will keep you dry (or dryer). However, the resulting aluminum chloride irritation takes a toll. Even if you aren't one of those whose armpits become immediately irritated and painful, the use of aluminum chloride keratinizes (hardens) the skin surface around the gland opening and leads to a gradual obstruction of the opening.

Depilatories are also very irritating and will cause a rash on anybody if left on long enough. Shaving powder is often resorted to to avoid the drawbacks of blade shaving. The powder, because of the sulfides it contains, usually has a terrible odor, which smells like rotten eggs. Sulfides and another ingredient called thioglycolate are both found in many depilatories, and they're both highly alkaline (detergent). They remove hair primarily by softening the surrounding skin, which dramatically lowers your reaction threshold. Almost anything can irritate unduly softened skin. Thioglycolates and sulfides are also frequently contained in permanent wave preparations. Solvents too are prime irritants. You'll get roughness or a rash as easily from nail polish remover as from soaking your hands in highly alkaline detergent!

Cosmetic Photosensitization

If it doesn't cause an allergic reaction, or a primary irritation, it just might give you a whale of a sunburn! Such is the unwelcome truth about numerous cosmetic formulas. Many ingredients are extremely photosensitizing, meaning they increase your potential to burn when exposed to sunshine. Oil of bergamot, for example, is contained in many perfumes and is a common cause of berlock dermatitis. This is a necklace of burns and rashes that appears on the necks of women who have patted on perfume before lying in the sun. What's worse, it leaves long-lasting dark blotches after the blisters have healed.

Lime essences are just as bad. Many vacationers return from the Caribbean with strange burns and blisters on the wrists and arms. They've simply sprayed themselves inadvertently with the lime wedges of poolside gin and tonic cocktails. The sun did the rest. Curiously, while lime is highly photosensitizing, lemon is completely safe.

Halogenated salicylanilides are the multisyllabic substances contained in deodorant soaps. In addition to their antiseptic properties, they are also very photosensitizing. Do not shower with a deodorant soap before a sunbath, or you'll look like a lobster in double time.

Further on I'm going to tell you about sunscreens and how to use them to protect your skin. But right here I want to point out that certain sunscreens actually cause a very rare incidence of photosensitization. Sunscreens that contain paba (para-aminobenzoic acid), the miracle ingredient described in Chapter 7, will ironically cause severe sunburns to isolated individuals.

Change of Pigment

Face powders very often contain coal tar derivatives. This causes hyperpigmentation, or darkening of the skin. You'll see many women whose necks and/or cheeks have become a little darker due to the powder they've been using.

Acne Cosmetica

All the moisturizers, foundations, liquids, lotions, powders, and whatnot are occlusive (clogging). They cover the skin and close up the pores. This traps the by-products of skin surface metabolism and leads to pimples and acne. Hypoallergenic cosmetics provide no additional protection against occlusion. There has been such a dramatic increase in adult acne that a new term, "acne cosmetica," has been added to the dermatologist's vocabulary. The occlusion that leads to acne is undoubtedly one of the worst side effects of cosmetics. For a fuller description of this, see Chapter 6.

Your skin is going to look much better once the damage already done by cosmetics has been corrected. You will be able to do that if you follow the regimens suggested in Chapter 1 and keep cosmetic usage to a bare minimum. Cosmetic manufacturers make much of their products' abilities to make you beautiful. Well, some of them actually do, at least temporarily. But the concept I want to get across here is that the use of cosmetic products presents unacceptable risks.

I offer the following concrete advice. You can give yourself a sensitivity test, and you should if you're bound and determined to use a cosmetic product regularly. Take a small amount of the product, rub it into the forearm, and leave it for twenty-four hours. Wait a week and do it again. Then wait another week and do it again. If there's no reaction in twelve to twenty-four hours, at least the product probably won't cause you to react allergically. Of course, if you do have a reaction like redness or rawness, don't use the stuff.

As for the "natural" products, they're baloney. Poison ivy is "natural" for that matter! Natural products can be just as allergenic, irritating, occlusive, photosensitizing, and so on as their chemically synthesized sisters.

The cosmetic that's hardest to go without, at least for the women who use it, is a moisturizer. Most available moisturizers either do nothing (like mouthwash), and vanish minutes after application, or they clog the pores with occlusive oils. Herewith, a formula for magic moisturizer that's guaranteed to work and costs only 50 cents! Take yourself to your local drugstore and buy a solution of hydrophilic petrolatum. The evening application is as follows. First soak the face with a warm wet towel for a few minutes. Pat dry and apply the medication. Repeat every night. This compound effectively seals in moisture better than almost anything on the market, although it is very occlusive.

Alternately, you can try a product that contains urea in a greaseless cream base. Urea is an aquaphilic; in other words, it chemically attracts water and tends to prevent its dissipation but doesn't clog the pores. Aquacare is a good product and comes in several strengths. Regular Aquacare contains 2 percent urea; Aquacare/HP (High Potency) has 10 percent urea. Another product, Carmol, contains 20 percent urea. While these moisturizers may contain a small percentage of lanolin, they also contain alcohol (a drying agent) and will not cause acne.

Chapter 6

Grown-up Acne

More than twenty million Americans suffer from some form of acne. As a group, they buy more prescription drugs than any other, thereby providing an enormous and lucrative market for the numerous pads, rubs, gels, and ointments that crowd the drugstore shelf. Some of these are excellent and others are quite worthless.

Acne is not exclusively a condition of adolescence. I regularly see young adults, particularly women in their twenties, and each asks virtually the same questions: "Is it something in my blood?" "Is there a hormone treatment to help me?" "Am I eating something that's causing this?" My aim in this chapter is to answer questions like these, and to tell you ways to clear up acne pimples.

First, I want to explain the basic concepts and define a few important terms. End organ sensitivity is the first of these, and it is the concept upon which rests the major medical approaches to the problem of acne. In this case, the end organ is the oil gland in the skin. If these oil glands are stimulated to produce excessive oil, an acnegenic (acne-prone) condition will exist. Hormones produced in the body, or ingested in medicines, stimulate the secretion of oil. And yet there may be two persons with the same blood level of hormones, but only one will have excessive oil secretion. Why? Simply because end organ sensitivity (in this case, the reaction of the oil gland to the presence of hormones) is entirely different from one individual to another. I can state this more simply by saying that some people get pimples, and some people don't.

A pustule is the official term for a pimple and it is the result of excessively oily skin. A whitehead is nothing more than a plugged-up oil gland whose surface opening is occluded (clogged) with excess sebum (oil). Left unattended, the sebaceous material clogging the gland will gradually become pigmented by melanin, the coloring protein produced by special cells in the oil gland. At this point, we call it a comedo (plural form, comedones). Squeezing—this will delight and surprise many—is emphatically recommended. By all means, go ahead and do it. The stories of society queens being reduced to tears when discovered squeezing a blackhead are utter nonsense. The pores are healthier for the cleaning.

However, unsuccessful or incorrect squeezing can sometimes cause a simple comedo to graduate into an unsightly red pimple filled with pus and surrounded with inflammation. The best way to squeeze is to buy a comedo extractor at a drugstore, nick off (de-roof) the top of the comedo with the pointed end, then press the hole in the small spoon end against the comedo.

Pus and redness are a result of chemical processes going on at skin level. The skin, like the other organs of the body, is host to a variety of normal bacteria, which in this case feed on the sebum produced by the sebaceous oil glands. In the process of metabolizing the oil, they produce fatty acids. As long as the skin is kept clean and the pores unclogged, irritating fatty acids won't even be noticed. However, if trapped too long within a comedo, either the fatty acids will by themselves leak through the walls of the oil gland and inflame the surrounding tissue, or the patient will squeeze the comedo improperly and actually force its contents into the surrounding tissue. This is extremely irritating and results in a rush of white blood cells (which comprise pus) to the site.

If sufficiently inflamed, the dermatologist will note that it has become a "jelly bean." These are just big, extremely inflamed pimples, whose lumps of pus we have all felt just below the skin level. Jelly beans are often caused hormonally, particularly in women just before the menstrual period. And this brings us to the role of hormones, specifically androgens, in acne.

As mentioned in Chapter 2, androgens are a family of hormones that have a clinically observable effect upon the skin. They make the oil glands grow. Testosterone (a male hormone produced in the testes) and progesterone (also a male-type hormone but produced by women, and contained in some birth-control pills) both contain androgens. So does cortisone, produced by the adrenal glands of both sexes and found in many medicines. When metabolized, the end products of these hormones will stimulate oil gland enlargement and the production of sebaceous oil. A person can prevent comedones by keeping the skin free of grease. Most drugstore products are for that purpose. But the condition of excessively oily or greasy skin has many unexpected causes.

The Major Causes of Acne

I'm going to tell you now about substances that are acnegenic. In and of themselves they will not cause pimples. They will, however, either induce a condition favorable to the formation of comedones (such as too much oil) or they are simply observed to have a high correlation with the incidence of acne.

Diet. It has long been impressed upon us that certain foods, usually oily foods, are responsible for acne. The ancients supposedly thought that blackheads were maggots feasting on the skin, and in fact "comedo" means "glutton" in Latin. Often the most delicious things are the most suspect. Take the following list for example:

chocolate
sugar
walnuts
candy
cheese
malted milk
oil- and deep-fried foods

Whatever the effect on the rest of the body of a diet heavy in the above substances, they have been shown to have no effect whatsoever on acne.

Chocolate in particular has been a traditional scapegoat. Its innocence was strongly suggested in an interesting experiment conducted in 1969 by a professor of dermatology. He and his co-workers were able to obtain a most unusual pair of chocolate bars. One bar had about twenty times the chocolate of the typical dime bar; the other had no chocolate whatsoever; to everyone's surprise, both bars tasted practically identical! The test continued for a period of a month on a total sample of sixty-five persons with moderate acne, of which thirty were adolescents and thirty-five were young male prison inmates in their twenties. The results were quite clear. The high amounts of chocolate had absolutely no effect on either the acne or the production of sebum. The experimenters themselves noted that many more experiments would doubtless have to be conducted and publicized before the public would accept conclusions that seem to fly in the face of long-accepted opinion.

Certain other edibles *are* known to be highly acnegenic. Sometimes it's because of androgen or androgen-like substances. Sometimes it's because of the presence of iodides and bromides. Both these latter can cause pustular reactions in the skin, although it's not specifically known why. But are there actually foods that cause acne? Yes, indeed! Health food diets, for instance, can ruin your skin. The following are particularly troublesome:

kelp (high iodide content)
seaweed (high iodide content)
sea salt (high iodide content)
saltwater fish (high iodide content)
wheat germ (high androgenic content)
wheat glutens (Gluten bread and meat substitutes made from glutens are both high-androgenic.)
cabbage (high iodide content)
shellfish (high idodide content)
spinach (high iodide content)
peanuts (high iodide content)
artichokes (high iodide content)
medicines that make you spit (cough medicines that contain iodides)
chain franchise fast foods (It's thought that the high iodide content of these burgers, fries, and so on results from the iodine used to disinfect the machinery that prepares them!)
multi-vitamins high in iodides or bromides
soft drinks with brominated vegetable oil or any other form of bromides

Hormones. Certain substances have been widely introduced into our food supply. One of the worst is the category of hormones known as steroids. Steroids are growth stimulators; ranchers, for example, dose their cattle considerably to encourage fast growth and weight gain. Unfortunately, steroids are acnegenic to a high degree. There are also studies correlating the introduction of steroids into the meat business with the increasing tendency for American men and women to become prematurely bald. Of course, these studies may or may not be true.

Just as you can improve acne by something as simple as changing the salt on your table (to a noniodized brand), women can sometimes radically improve an acne condition by changing birth-control pills. Bear in mind that there is no specific age for acne. It has to do with hormone levels and can occur at any age. Sometimes I see thirty-year-old women breaking out like teen-agers because they're using the wrong birth-control pill. Those containing progesterone will cause some women to have acne. Estrogen-loaded pills are often much better, despite such side effects as breast enlargement or headaches.

Medicines. Many medications cause acne. Bromides, which are highly acnegenic, are found in literally hundreds of over-the-counter drug products. The cortisone in poison-ivy treatments is acnegenic. Nurses in tubercular wards often use a drug called INH, which counters tuberculosis but is also acnegenic. Likewise are the iodides contained in many cough and cold medicine formulas. Another unexpected source is the phenobarbitol in diet pills and in drugs widely used by asthma sufferers. Dilantin, used by literally millions of Americans for seizure problems, can cause pimples too.

You can't imagine how many people are unwittingly giving themselves acne. A simple way to tell if you're one of them is to observe whether the condition is "monolesional" (all whiteheads or all blackheads or all jelly beans). If so, it's 90 percent certain that these pimples have sprung from the same cause, very likely some substance you've introduced into yourself.

Acne Cosmetica. Myth: Makeup has no effect on the skin. Wrong! Women's magazines won't offend their advertisers and tell you the truth. Namely, that cosmetics are occlusive (pore-clogging) and often contain acnegenic oils. To simply stop using makeup will often clear the face completely. But the woman who degreases the skin, opens the pores, lets out the trapped fatty acids, clears her skin, and then goes right back to using the occlusive cosmetic will quickly get pimples again.

Beware of moisturizing foundations, at least those that do not contain urea (see Chapter 5). While they will saturate the skin with oil and temporarily banish wrinkles, they will also usually cause pimples. As a general rule, when you're young, it's better to have dry skin. The skin's tolerance for oils increases with age. Cold creams are great for grandmothers. Young women should stick to Ivory. Don't bother with soaps that contain coconut oil or goat's milk, natural herbs, oranges or bananas. They're all baloney. Somebody who recently came to me was using a soap filled with vitamin E. She was paying $4 a bar and getting a faceful of pimples without knowing why. Like the oil in moisturizing creams, vitamin E oil is acnegenic when applied topically. If you're acne-prone at all, keep away from any oil product that does not contain urea. And use brush-on blushers, rather than pots of gloss on your cheeks.

Men should beware of pomade acne, clusters of closely set comedones on the forehead. The oil and impure ingredients in cheap hair grooming aids are almost always the cause.

Perioral Dermatitis. In recent years dermatologists have noted a great increase of young women with a new and baffling complaint. The symptoms resemble regular acne, although they usually consist of pustules and pimples around the mouth and on the chin. At first dermatologists treated this condition like acne but with very disappointing results. Regular acne medicines usually made it worse. Gradually it evolved that they were dealing with a different condition.

There is a continuing debate over what, exactly, perioral dermatitis is, but some interesting findings have been obtained: (1) Sometimes, it's actually a yeast infection; (2) the fluorinated steroid creams for treating rashes and eczema will make the condition worse; and (3) the only treatment that consistently improves the situation is a very mild, bland cream containing anti-yeast agents. The cure lies in recognizing an often confusing condition.

Heredity. If your parents had pimples, you probably do too. Simply because your end organ sensitivity level is something that is genetically inherited.

Acne Can Cause Scars

People get pimples everywhere—behind the ears, in the armpits, in the groin. It's a matter of where you're oily. But the worst kind are those that disfigure the face. Bad cases of acne can scar a face permanently, unless there's proper dermatological care during crisis attacks.

There are three types of acne scars. Keloids are raised scars; pockmarks are depressed scars; and ice-pick scars are long, deep holes that often go sideways into the skin.

A keloid results as a hyper-reaction to a trauma on the skin—like a big infected pimple. There is a treatment for keloids consisting of intralesional injections of steroids. This means actually injecting medication into the scar. The steroids cause keloid tissue to shrink. Susceptibility to keloids is largely genetic. Some people scar more easily than others. For instance, many black men are plagued by razor bumps, which are keloids caused by shaved hairs that have curled back into the flesh and plugged an oil gland. First comes a big pimple, then comes the keloid.

Pockmarks and ice-pick scars are treated differently. One method, called dermabrasion, consists of a fast circular sander that actually grinds down the epidermis surrounding the pitted scar in an effort to level the skin surface. This method, while widely practiced, comes with no guarantees. It may require repeated treatments, and then might even make you look worse. If the dermis is injured by a careless operator, the result can be a bad scar. And if none of the above happens, there's a chance that the new layers of epidermis that replace those sanded away will be either hyper- or hypopigmented (lighter or darker colored than the rest of you).

Alternately, there's chemabrasion, wherein a strong inflammatory solution is applied to the skin so as to peel off the top layers. Sometimes this peels the holes off too. Sometimes it results in the same problems of scarring, pigmentation, and unsatisfactory results. For further discussion of dermabrasion and chemabrasion, see Chapter 14.

Scar treatments are, however, effective to a certain extent, and it can be said that the worse you look, the more dramatic the improvement is likely to be. Results of therapy for mild cases of scarring are not so encouraging. Good care from the beginning avoids bad scars.

What to Do If You Have Acne

1. Determine the cause accurately. Before you dash off to the doctor, ask yourself the following questions.

"Am I under undue stress?" Very often stressful periods lead to outbreaks of acne. If you're in the middle of one, get some extra sleep and calm down.

"Is there a relationship between acne and my menstrual period?" If there seems to be, see your gynecologist. Possibly you should change to a different type of birth-control pill.

"Have I started any new medications?" Drugs like cortisone, for example, cause acne as a side effect. Perhaps your doctor will taper your dosage or switch you to a different medication.

"Have I changed my makeup?" Possibly you should cut out makeup altogether and use an astringent like Seba-Nil to counter the acnegenic oils contained in almost all makeups. Seba-Nil has acetone, alcohol, and water, which combine very effectively to dry the skin.

"Have I been out in the sun lately?" Sunshine, especially on that midwinter jaunt to the Caribbean, tends to initially draw out whiteheads. Abrasive scrubs like Pernox will peel the top layer of skin and usually relieve the problem. Acne soaps with salicylic acid will do the same. Good ones are Fostex and SAStid.

"Am I eating acnegenic food?" Maybe you are. Refer to our list at the beginning of this chapter.

2. Over-the-Counter Medications. Conventional therapy for acne basically boils down to drying up the skin. There are a host of products on the market, many of which are not very useful. When shopping, look for

ingredients like precipitated sulfur, resorcinol, and especially benzoyl peroxide. Good products include:

Benoxyl
Transact
Rezamid
Xerac
Thera-Blem
Acnomel
Fostex

If you have light skin and eyes, you might want to try something a little milder, like Klaron or Rezamid.

An excellent over-the-counter product is Vanoxide. The active ingredient is benzoyl peroxide, which is mildly irritating and causes good peeling. When you first begin to use it, make it half-strength, so it's not as irritating. This way the skin won't get too dry.

Individual skins react variably to individual products. My advice is to buy more than one product and experiment. Always be sure to read the labels and follow directions closely. A further piece of advice is to start out with only one application per day. No matter what the label says, start slowly.

Many of these products are colorless and can be matched to your complexion by your pharmacist's color blender. Again I must warn dark-skinned readers that products containing resorcinol will cause dark staining of the skin.

Acne soaps are another excellent way to degrease the skin. Stiefel Laboratories makes about twenty different types, among them SAStid and Acne-Aid. These antiseptic soaps are abrasive enough to remove the top layer of the skin, taking the oil gland plugs along with it. They're also very cheap.

Excessive oil and grease can cause pimples anywhere.

Workers in oil refineries can get them behind their knees! People with oily hair often break out along the hairline. Even if your acne is not limited to hairline areas, an acne shampoo is extremely helpful if you have oily hair. Westwood Laboratories makes both an abrasive soap containing polyethyline granules and a drying anti-dandruff shampoo marketed under the name Pernox. However, almost any anti-dandruff shampoo will usually dry adequately.

Your skin might also respond well to more abrasive soaps containing sand and silicates, like Brāsivol whose particles come in small, medium, and large. Komex is another good one with an unusual formula containing particles that dissolve completely. The way to use these soaps is to work up a rich lather with hot water, rinse, repeat, and towel-dry, leaving the medication on to do its work. Extra-strong products are in gel form, like Desquam-X5, PanOxyl-5 Gel, and PanOxyl-10 Gel.

Squeezing Pimples

There is a right way and wrong way to do it. The danger, of course, is that you will force those highly irritating fatty acids into the surrounding tissue. Result: a big, red pimple. Cosmetologists and dermatologists do it just fine, usually with the aid of what's called a comedo extractor (available at many pharmacies for around $2). One end is pointed and is used to loosen the oil plug. The other end is rather like a tiny spoon with a hole in the middle. Press the hole over the whitehead or blackhead and squeeze slightly to the side. Be sure to clean the skin and the instrument when you're finished. Alternately, you can loosen the plug (de-roof it) with a pin and squeeze with the fingers.

Don't squeeze in the "triangle of death." This ominously titled area is a triangle on the face whose top point lies roughly between the eyebrows and lower points are just above the corners of the mouth, thus encompassing the area on either side of the nose. Now I know perfectly well that every one of you has had a pimple there, has squeezed it, and is living to read this page. Nevertheless, the veins from this particular region drain into what's called the cavernous sinus, located beneath the brain. An infection in the cavernous sinus can be fatal. And while it isn't common, it's a condition that's not all that rare. So beware.

Licensed cosmetologists will squeeze all your pimples quite professionally. For around $12, a cosmetologist will spend fifty minutes on you and you alone. Look in the yellow pages, remembering that many localities arrange their yellow pages differently. If you can't find a listing under cosmetologists, try "facials" or "beauty treatments." Beware of quacks; be sure you go to someone who has a state license in cosmetology.

Sunshine. While the sun will often cause an initial outbreak of whiteheads, its long-range effect is extremely beneficial. Almost everybody's acne is better in the summer because of increased exposure to sunshine. A sunlamp is good too, but sunshine is the best.

What Can Doctors Do About Acne?

A major role of any dermatologist is to prescribe appropriate antibiotic medication. The number one prescribed drug is tetracycline, which is taken the wrong way by 90 percent of the people who take it.

The usual problem is underdosage. But even if the

patient takes enough, he is seldom advised to take it at least an hour before or after meals. Tetracycline binds to calcium and will pass right out of the system if combined with any calcium in your meal. Among the side effects of this drug is a tendency to cause upset stomach. And patients who take Tums or Gelusil for the stomach will again cause the tetracycline to bind to the calcium in those products and exit from the system. It's because of the reaction with calcium that the drug is not recommended for growing children or pregnant women (it can turn the teeth of babies green!) Tetracycline also supresses normal bacteria and allows yeast to come to the surface. The result in women is a high incidence of yeast infections.

For all this, the drug works exceedingly well. It is bacteriostatic instead of bacteriocidal, meaning that it lets the skin bacteria live but changes their metabolism. The chains of fatty acids produced by bacteria in the presence of tetracycline are simply not so inflammatory. Penicillin actually does this job even better. However, since penicillin is not fat soluble, it can't even get into the oil gland where the action is and so is useless against acne.

The most commonly prescribed pill contains about 250 milligrams of tetracycline. You should take from three to four per day. Often people are too impatient for results. A six- to eight-month course is often needed to properly clear the acne. There is no difference in quality between name-brand tetracycline and the house brands offered by big drug chains. Buy the house brand, which is always substantially less expensive.

Second generation tetracyclines, recently introduced on the market, are unnecessarily strong. So are the side effects. Minocycline and Declomycin are examples, and for most people, they're not worth the extra risk or money. However, they can be effective in refractory cases.

Any tetracycline used in conjunction with birth-control pills may cause a yeast infection. A home solution is to change the pH of the vagina with a do-it-yourself douche containing one part vinegar and two parts water. In an era of spray-on, flesh-flavoring cosmetics, this is not going to be the solution for everyone. Alternately, there is a product called Mysteclin-F, which combines tetracycline with an anti-yeast agent.

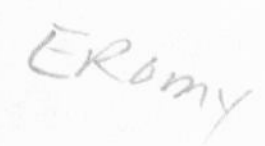

Your dermatologist may choose an entirely different approach to your acne problem, and prescribe a bacteriocidal agent such as erythromycin. This is a second-line drug that kills the bacteria that produce the irritating fatty acids. The side effects are few, although some people do get terrible stomach cramps. Erythromycin usually passes through the body quickly and smoothly, even more so if taken with a container of yogurt.

Problem acne will sometimes respond paradoxically. Hydrocortisone, for example, is a steroid that would seem to be acnegenic (since cortisone is). But there are times when a short treatment will clear up acne that simply will not respond to anything else.

Doctors can also employ any of several topical approaches. There's a lot of show biz surrounding injections of intralesional steroids, such as Kenelog, directly into the pimple; and results are amazingly fast. Prescription acne gels of pure benzoyl peroxide are highly inflammatory, but they effectively strip off the top layer of skin and dramatically open clogged pores. If you're a patient who really likes to see things happening, your doctor might try liquid nitrogen or dry ice. Again, this treatment removes the top layer of skin, albeit not too delicately.

Some doctors persist in using X rays, but many of us are leery of this treatment. During the Depression years,

X rays were widely used to counteract fungus infections on the scalp. Many young boys underwent these treatments, which were also used against ringworm infections. Thirty-five years later there was a frighteningly high incidence of premature baldness, skin cancer on the scalp, even insanity. Taking into further account the ever-present danger of overdose, I think this treatment extremely unwise unless in expert hands.

There's a new product out called RETIN-A. This is vitamin A acid and is not to be confused with the vitamin A we take orally. It comes in three forms: wash-and-drys, cream, and liquid. RETIN-A hardens the top layer of the epidermis. This means that it hardens the skin, where the oil is normally secreted, to the point where comedo formation virtually stops. Thus the very cause of acne can be alleviated. The effect is rapidly reversible, so the product must be used religiously. It shouldn't be applied to open pustules, which most adults don't have anyway. If used daily, it will eliminate whiteheads and blackheads often without resort to antibiotics.

RETIN-A is often especially powerful in conjunction with other products. Used with tetracycline, it's fantastically effective. Likewise, it is particularly potent with Vanoxide. It really works, but you must use it every day.

There are drawbacks. RETIN-A may be overly drying, the liquid and swab forms especially. It also tends to make things look a bit horrible at first. Whiteheads will become jelly-like and slushy before they disappear. This product is also extremely photosensitizing, and the unwarned user might get a particularly bad sunburn in no time. If your doctor doesn't warn you about this photosensitization, get another doctor!

As of this writing, the Food and Drug Administration is still considering approval of revolutionary new products manufactured by the Upjohn Company. Prostaglandins, as they are called, are mediators of inflammation that have a strong anti-lipase (fat) activity. They seem, so far, to dramatically diminish pimples. More tests will be needed before they're prescribed, so this is just a preview of news to come.

Chapter 7

The Sun, Sports, and Your Skin

The sun is not nearly so dangerous as popular belief would have it. The sun emits a wide spectrum of wavelengths, but only certain ones concern us. These particular wavelengths are dangerous and can cause chromosomal damage. The earth's atmosphere contains enough carbon dioxide, water, and ozone to shield us here on the surface, at least until the SST depletes the ozone layer.

Suntans (and sunburns) are the result of skin exposure to a specific range of wavelengths. Numerous rays fall within this range, only some of which will tan, while others do nothing more than burn. The old myth that you must get a burn in order to tan is just that—an old myth.

Why do people get sunburned? The burn is localized skin injury resulting from excess exposure to ultraviolet sunrays. Blood vessels in the exposed skin will dilate and cause increased blood flow (vasodilatation), and the increased flow leads to increased permeability of the blood vessel walls. This combines with the disintegration of small enzyme packets called lysosomes. Ultraviolet rays will cause these packets, which are contained in all cells, to burst apart, thereby releasing irritating enzymes. The irritation and the increased blood flow combine to cause the redness and edema (fluid collection and swelling) that characterize sunburn.

Sunburns will show up as an initial faint redness that curiously disappears quickly. Then two to four hours will elapse before pain and redness flood the skin again, with much more strength. The burn will peak within fourteen to twenty hours and usually persist from one to two full days.

Suntans are caused by increased dispersion of melanin, the protein complex contained in the skin that produces color. Too many sunburns and/or too much tanning cause undue wrinkling, atrophy of the skin tissue, and solar elastosis. This last item is the term for the degeneration of the elastic tissue within the skin, the sagging that happens when sun exposure is excessive. None of this is necessary, thanks to the excellent sunscreen products now on the market.

Choosing the Right Sunscreen

It is not difficult to tan without burning. You only need the right sunscreen. The miracle ingredient to look for in any sunscreen product is para-aminobenzoic acid, or more simply paba. Paba works best in an alcohol lotion vehicle, and ideally you should apply it about forty-five minutes before going into the sun. What it does is bind to the horny layer of the skin, thereby deflecting dangerous burning rays. Despite label claims, it will wash off in a tennis sweat or after a dip in the pool, so keep reapplying. Paba products are easily obtainable over-the-

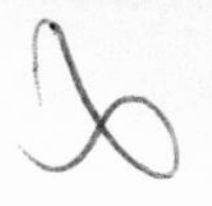

counter. My favorites are PreSun and Eclipse, both big brands widely sold. Paba is a clear yellow substance that tends to stain light-colored nylons and so on, so be careful. Cinnamates, derived from cinnamon oil, are also excellent screeners of dangerous sunrays. But in my opinion, paba products are definitely superior.

Sunscreens will selectively screen out redness-producing rays. Sun-blockers will screen out everything. The best blocker is zinc oxide paste, sold over-the-counter for people who can't tolerate any exposure at all. This is the stuff that looks like war paint on your nose. If even more protection is needed, a paba sunscreen plus a titanium dioxide paste will block anything short of a punch in the nose. Your druggist will have to make up the titanium paste for you.

Beneficial Effects of the Sun

Aside from making the world go 'round, the sun has a most salutory effect on acne. Sunlight encourages a rapid reproduction of skin tissue, which in turn causes a peeling of the epidermis. As the top epidermal layer peels off, it unblocks pores and opens comedones.

The dry and scaly skin condition known as eczema typically improves in the summer, because of increased exposure to sunshine. Likewise, the media's famous "heartbreak" of psoriasis improves with exposure to sunshine. In fact, the most advanced treatment for bad cases of psoriasis consists of artificially inducing a bad sunburn. Treatments of this sort have recently been carried out at Massachusetts General Hospital, where phototoxic chemicals were applied to patients sitting under black (ultraviolet) light. The terrible sunburn that results leads not only to peeling, but also will retard cell turnover time, the unnatural rapidity of which is the cause of psoriasis.

In lieu of the sun itself, sufferers of any of the above conditions, or healthy people who want a tan, should all avail themselves of sunlamps. These lamps should be used with extreme caution. The General Electric 275 RS is probably the most popular sunlamp on the market. It emits one wavelength only, a 2537 angstrom model, by means of low-pressure mercury vapor. It is excellent and easily obtainable even in drugstores.

First, be sure your eyes are shielded with opaque goggles. They usually come with the lamp, but if they don't, be sure to buy a pair. Next, be certain to avoid excess exposure initially. Start out with five seconds only. Yes that's right. Five seconds only. Increase your exposure by five more seconds each day. When you hit a golden brown, keep that level. Follow this procedure and you'll never get burned. The tan you get will not fade easily either.

The distance you sit from the lamp really depends on the size of the bulb. Follow the manufacturer's directions. And remember that whereas sunlamps are good, there is no substitute for the real thing.

What's Bad About the Sun?

First let's differentiate between phototoxic and photoallergic. Phototoxicity can affect everybody and anybody. It describes a condition of excessive dosage either of sunshine alone or sunshine plus some toxic chemical that together cause a bad reaction. For instance, normal sun exposure is good for you, but excessive sun is toxic—it causes a burn. Oil of bergamot in a perfume base won't hurt you, but in combination with sunshine it is phototoxic—it causes a burn. Similarly, second generation tetracyclines prescribed for acne will cause phototoxic reactions in the sunshine. Usually hyperpigmentation (darkening of the skin) is the legacy of a phototoxic reaction. These reactions do not manifest themselves uniformly among all of us. Phototoxic reactions like rashes, burns, and edema (swelling) are governed equally by our individual tolerances as well as by degree of dosage.

Photoallergic responses are less common and usually harder to diagnose. Whereas a toxic substance or combination will cause damage in and of itself, photoallergic responses only happen to people who are specifically allergic to a combination of the sun and something else. For example, Thiazide water pills that treat blood pressure will cause allergic reactions only among people who are allergic to the pill plus sunshine. It's not a matter of dose, but of sensitization. Many oral diabetic drugs cause photoallergic reactions, as do some tranquilizers and griseofulvin (a drug used to treat fungal infections). Oftentimes the photoallergic reaction is delayed, and sometimes it extends to areas that weren't even exposed to the sun, which further compounds the problem of correct diagnosis. Many conditions that are thought to be eczema are actually photoallergic reactions.

Furocoumarins are a family of chemical substances notable for phototoxicity. They include a surprising list: oil of bergamot (in many perfumes), lime (in perfumes and flavorings), parsnip, fennel, dill, parsley, carrots, and celery are all furocoumarins. Whether you ingest them or rub them on the skin's surface, they are phototoxic. Your reaction, of course, depends on the dose. Ironically, many natural cosmetics and herb soaps contain furocoumarins that cause terrible sunburns, especially preparations made from lime or carrots.

The word cancer is enough to send shivers of dread through anybody (see also Chapter 11). Skin cancer, however, is possibly the blandest and least dangerous cancer around. It is a condition of uncontrolled proliferation of skin growth, and as such, it resembles other cancers. However, it is very rarely fatal and usually doesn't look like more than a brownish discoloration or a case of acne. It will not spread to other organs of the body either. There is a higher incidence of skin cancer among people who work outdoors. Nowadays, paba sunscreens are being used prophylactically among outdoor workers to help prevent this problem.

The vast majority of people aren't troubled by skin cancer. But the cumulative effect of too much sun over a lifetime is not good. The sun's rays will slowly destroy collagen and elastin, two important proteins contained in lower levels of the dermis. Collagen is called the backbone of the skin, and if it's lost or damaged, the result is wrinkles. Elastin provides tone and body, without which the skin will sag and droop. Let me stress that destruction of these two proteins is a cumulative process that entails many years of overexposure.

Sunshine may also interact with elements of your environment in a deleterious manner. Pregnant women exposed to excessive sunlight will often develop chloasma, a hormonal reaction that causes brown blotches on the cheeks. The effect of birth-control pills, estrogen and progesterone types alike, is to simulate pregnancy, so chloasma can also affect women who might not be pregnant but who are taking birth-control pills. It's possible that you are taking other medicines that are photosensitizing (either phototoxic or photoallergic).

Without realizing it, you can get an excruciating sunburn from relatively little exposure. Here is a list of seven substances to be most wary of:

Thiazide Diuretics. It is not known why the ingestion of Thiazide, prescribed for high blood pressure, leads to photosensitization, but it does. If you take this medication, you must be particularly wary of the sun.

Oral Hypoglycemics. These are anti-diabetic drugs, and millions of people take them. In fact, almost half the population of this country suffers from either high blood pressure or diabetes. A great percentage of these people are under medication that can cause very bad sunburns.

Saccharin. Very photosensitizing, as are most artificial sweeteners.

Thorazine. Very photosensitizing, as are many tranquilizers.

Halogenated Salicylanilides. This is the active ingredient in deodorant soaps. It is so photosensitizing that hotels and motels throughout the southern states have stopped equipping guest rooms with antibacterial soaps, lest unwary guests at poolside be burned to a crisp.

Oil of Bergamot. Berlock dermatitis is the term for the neck ring of rashes and burns some women develop after a sunbath. The condition results from perfume being applied around the neck. Most perfumes contain oil of bergamot, a highly photosensitizing substance.

Essences of Lemon and Lime. Citric essences are enjoying a great vogue these days and crop up in everything from after-shave to bath soap to Mr. Clean. Limes are highly photosensitizing, so beware. Even a stray squirt from a poolside cocktail can cause a painful burn or rash if exposed to the sun.

Sunshine has a few other obscure bad points. It can make certain rare diseases worse. Lupus erythematosus is a case in point. Do you have rashes in unlikely locations (on top of the hands? on the face except under the chin?); if so, you may be a lupus sufferer and not even know it! Perhaps you've fallen victim to Majorca acne. This condition was observed among young Scandinavian females who vacationed in Spain and returned home with terrible cases of acne. Well, sometimes for reasons unknown, sudden sun exposure will bring out an unexpected case of pimples. Similarly, the herpes virus that causes those uncomfortable blisters on the lips and/or genitals can be exacerbated by sunlight.

A Special Regimen for Skin Care in the Sun

I started this chapter telling you that sunshine can be beneficial. The four simple steps that follow will practically guarantee the suntan you've always wanted, with attendant salutory effects on acne and other skin conditions.

Begin Sun Exposure Slowly. I've told you about sunlamps and how to use them. If you're going to a tropical resort, your first day should involve no more than fifteen minutes in the sun. Increase sun dosage slowly and you won't get fried. You can prepare for a southern vacation by starting your tan under a sunlamp.

Use Sunscreens That Contain Paba. This ingredient really works against potentially burning rays. And despite the label claims on PreSun and Eclipse, paba does not retard tanning. I advise patients to reapply it continually and liberally, every fifteen minutes during a sunbath.

Avoid Deodorant Soaps. They can cause severe sunburns.

Apply Moisturizers at Night. Remember that acne-prone people should use products containing urea. These include Aquacare, Aquacare/HP, and Carmol. Older women can use oilier products. Aquaphore is a good one; it's actually a fancy Vaseline. Eucerin is good too; it contains the ingredients of Aquaphore plus water and perfume. Nivea is also excellent. If dry skin is a regular problem, you are advised to wash with an oil soap like Oilatum during the sunbathing season.

In addition to the sun, there are several other natural factors, found in their most potentially dangerous combinations in the area of athletics, that can be enemies of healthy skin.

Wind. When combined with hot sun, exposure to a strong wind will intensify the aforementioned sun reactions. Why this is so is not fully understood. Some suggest that a continual wind tends to disguise how hot you really become. This makes post-exposure hydration doubly important.

Sweat. An overheated body engaged in pitched athletic contest can literally sweat so much it all can't get out. This leads to the troublesome sweat retention syndrome, which is frequently (though not exclusively) stress related. Miliaria is the name for a condition that often occurs among people who'll spend an entire Saturday with a shirt stuck wetly to their backs. Miliaria are little bump-like blisters on the back filled with sweat that can't get out. It's itchy and irritating, and it probably means that you should take it a little easier. ZeaSORB is a good OTC (over-the-counter) powder that aids drying. Calamine Lotion is good for the condition too, in that it has a mild drying action that will de-roof the multiple milia. You can have the sweaty sock syndrome too. This is characterized by huge, irritating, sweat-filled blisters on the foot. Again, ZeaSORB helps, as does prophylactic use of deodorant foot sprays.

Water. Water tends to dehydrate the skin, whether or not combined with sun exposure. Remember this, and remember to hydrate the skin with a cool bath and a hydrating preparation (like Aquacare) after water exposure. Salt water combined with sun will often have a particularly salutory effect on eczema, psoriasis, and a host of rare dermatological conditions. The Dead Sea, incidentally, is a great mecca for psoriasis sufferers, who often display dramatic improvements.

Cold. Most people who think they've had frostbite have actually endured a case of chilblains. This first cousin to frostbite is curiously more common among women than men. It consists of blue to black discolorations on the skin from long exposure to the cold. Even after you come indoors, the discoloration can linger. What to do? Try a hypopigmenting agent such as ammoniated mercury or any of the bleaching creams that contain hydroquinone. Many OTC products contain these ingredients.

What you really should do is avoid becoming so cold. It's dehydrating at best. At worst, you may have to contend with frostbite, in which the skin of the extremities literally freezes. There are differing opinions on how best to treat frozen toes and noses, but most doctors advise that the affected areas be warmed extremely slowly.

Some Common Sports-Related Skin Conditions

Blisters. A blister is a separation of the epidermis from the dermis. It's caused when the skin is traumatized, either by walking, rowing, or any number of sports. Sunburns will cause a similar trauma, as will many chemical burns, diabetes, and a host of rare skin diseases.

The physical trauma that pulls the skin layers apart also liberates certain chemicals in the skin, which cause blood vessels to leak. What comes out of the leaky vessel and into the blister is a clear liquid called edema fluid, or serum. Why isn't it red? Because red blood cells are just too big to leak through blood vessel walls, even under these conditions of increased permeability.

As long as the blister remains closed, chances are it will remain sterile. So if it doesn't hurt and/or isn't too big, I say leave it alone. If the blister must be punctured, the trick is not to let it happen spontaneously. Open blisters are prone to bacterial infection, which is easy to avoid. Some doctors suggest that you sterilize a pin over a flame and pierce the blister twice. Like a can of beer, it needs two holes to drain properly. Apply an OTC antibacterial ointment such as Bacitracin on the pinholes, flatten the skin on top, and cover with a Band-Aid.

Callouses. A callous is just a different response to the same traumas that cause blisters. Constant trauma of tremendous walking, orthopedic bone problems, bad shoes, too much running, handling of objects, or whatever will cause skin on the affected area to thicken.

However, you may actually have a wart and not a callous. Most people can't tell the difference. Here's an easy test to tell which is which. When you press straight down on a corn or a callous it hurts. But if you squeeze it, it doesn't hurt. Conversely, pressing straight down on a wart is painless; but squeezing it is quite painful. This is handy knowledge especially for the feet, where warts and callouses can look exactly the same.

The treatment for callouses is to physically remove them. The best idea for people with corns and callouses is to go to a podiatrist. If you've never been to one, get ready for a sensual treat. It's cheap, painless, and you'll feel ten pounds lighter. Alternately, you can pick, grind, or rub them off yourself. Pumice stones help many people, but a chiropody sponge works even better. These are hard, curiously textured little sponges that work quite amazingly. The Heros company makes a good one.

Other treatments include shaving them off yourself with a razor, which is all right if you don't mind a little bleeding. You might also buy an OTC 40 percent salicylic acid plaster from your druggist and keep it taped over the callous for a week. When it's uncovered, the hard tissue will have become white and spongy. You can scrape off the detritus, and apply another plaster if necessary.

Poison Ivy. The medical term is rhus dermatitis, rhus being the irritating chemical in the ivy's sap. For campers who don't know already, poison ivy grows low and has a characteristic triple cluster of waxy reddish-green leaves with pointed tips. Even after the growing season, enough rhus can remain in partially shriveled leaves to give you a bad case. That's why so many people get it after raking fall leaves.

Poison ivy is characterized by large grouped blisters on a red base surrounded by a halo of redness. It's a question whether or not it's contagious. But the reaction is caused by the presence of rhus and not by the blisters themselves. I don't like most of the topical OTC medicines, since they contain antihistamines and often cause allergic responses. The best treatment is a simple home remedy. First wash with brown laundry soap, then apply cool compresses soaked in a half-and-half mixture of water and skim milk. If the disease continues to spread, see a dermatologist for some systemic medication to accompany the compresses. If you do get pills (they're usually oral steroids), be sure to keep taking them for at least three weeks. Too many people note early improvement, stop the medication, and suffer what's called the bounce-back phenomenon: namely, a renewed worsening of the condition.

One of the classic growth spots for poison ivy is cemeteries. Every September, after Jewish high holy days and cemetery visits, my office is flooded with Jewish poison ivy victims. "But, Doctor, I live on Eighty-fourth Street! How can I get poison ivy?" is the common refrain. Then there are times when it's not cemetery ivy either, but what's called cemetery rash. This afflicts many city dwellers who are often exposed to the first sun of the season while visiting a grave. It's a phototoxic reaction caused by the combination of some foodstuff or drug in the system with unexpected sun. The resulting rash and blisters often look just like poison ivy.

Bugs. Camping out or just lounging on the lawn carries the built-in hazard of bug bites, and there's not much you can do about it. Insects are often drawn by the scent of sweat. Insect repellents help at times, but they often cause allergic reactions.

Bug bites are not always recognized as such. But any time you see grouped lesions on the skin without an obvious cause, think bugs. These lesions are papules, and each has a central punctum where the bite occurred. A papule is like a little hive; it's your body's reaction to whatever the bug pumped into you. They're grouped because bugs typically bite several times.

The simplest thing to do with insect bites is to apply witch hazel or rubbing alcohol. Depending on severity, your doctor might recommend a topically applied steroid cream. And if you're getting married tomorrow and have a huge mosquito bite on your nose, your doctor can also make an intralesional steroid injection right into the bite. This will make it go away in less than a day.

Tennis Toe. A toenail that suddenly turns black has frightened many a tennis or squash player. Why? Because it's sometimes a symptom of cancerous malignant melanoma. Fortunately, it's also a symptom of a much more benign condition called tennis toe.

The cause of tennis toe is nothing more than short stops on the tennis court, or the jogging track, or whatever, that traumatize the toenails. The result is a hematoma (blood hemorrhage) under the nail. This very often happens after the first game of the season. If it has happened to you, just watch the pigmented area and note whether it moves out with growth. If it does, you're OK; if not, you might be in trouble (see Chapter 12).

Jock Itch. Rashes in the groin (jock itch) are extremely common and have three main causes. Unfortunately, any given case may well stem from a combination of these causes.

The first is called intertrigo. This is a rash caused by sweating thighs rubbing together. It often shows up after sports, involves no pathogen, and typically afflicts people with overweight thighs. If this is you, dispense immediately with jockey shorts or bikini pants and change to well-powdered boxer shorts. You can soothe the rash itself either with Calamine Lotion or with an old standby called Castellani's paint. The Italians knighted Castellani for this discovery during the last war, when jock itch descended on the Italian army invading Ethiopia. His paint (still very much in use) is red in color, tends to smart a bit, and will stain everything. It is cheap, however, and even mildly anti-fungal and anti-monilial (yeast).

The second major cause of jock itch is fungus infection. You can tell when the rash is fungally induced if the central area of the rash is clear, while the border has bumps and is active. Active borders are typical of fungus infections. Tinactin is a good, safe, OTC anti-fungal product available in cream, liquid, and powder. Apply the cream or liquid to the rash, and again switch to boxer shorts or step-ins liberally dusted with Tinactin powder.

Monilial (yeast) infections are the third major cause of jock itch. This time, there's a rash in the groin accompanied by the appearance of satellite lesions and pustules in outlying areas of the thighs. The treatment is again to dry it up with powder or Castellani's paint. Or, your doctor can prescribe an anti-yeast agent such as Nystatin.

Swimmer's Itch. Many lakes in the United States are inhabited by a bug called schistasome. A frequently observed reaction occurs in swimmers who use these waters. They get little infestations of schistasome larvae in the skin of the elbows, which then spread to the arms causing red papules that itch like crazy. Unfortunately, there's no good treatment available. The best preventative is just to towel yourself vigorously after swimming.

Swimming Pool Granuloma. This happens in pools that aren't clean. Specifically, you'll get a small cut or scrape or graze from diving or horseplay, and the next thing you know a lump begins to grow. The lump is a reaction to a specific bacteria, which incidentally is closely related to TB. The cure is local destruction, either by cutting, burning, or freezing. Once destroyed, the granuloma won't return. Sometimes, the TB medicine called INH is prescribed. It works well on the granuloma but causes acne as a side effect.

Sand Rash. This condition, which looks terrible, consists of perifollicular (around the hair follicles) hemorrhages. It's caused by abrasive beach sand in wet crotches and goes away all by itself after giving you a good scare!

Windburn. The dry, red, scaly, or flaky skin that often accompanies undue wind exposure is the result of dehydration. Creams won't avoid it. What you need is an ointment that clings, and lots of it. Wind and sun together form a double threat of dehydration.

Chapped Lips. Again, it's a case of dehydration caused by sun, wind, cold, or any combination thereof. To avoid it, you need a physical barrier. Chapstick is good, since it's an ointment. Even more effective is zinc oxide ointment or paste. You'll look like a clown, but your lips won't get chapped! Alternately, good glossy lipsticks are excellent protection. What's important is keeping the barrier constantly on the lips, especially the lower lip, which is most exposed to the elements.

Chapter 8

Lines and Wrinkles: What You Can Do Now to Avoid Them Later

Everybody's going to age and get weathered on their voyage through life. To that extent, lines and wrinkles are inevitable. However, many times it happens prematurely. To understand when you can do what, about which ones, please note that wrinkles come in two basic varieties: Some wrinkles are permanent, and some wrinkles aren't. To rid the face of the permanent type requires radical plastic surgery. The non-permantnt types—pseudowrinkles I call them—are relatively easy to banish.

Pseudowrinkles are really nothing more than the effect of dehydration on the skin. But they often look just like the permanent lines and wrinkles of age and cause just as much concern. They result from very ordinary situations, five of which follow:

Five Major Causes of Pseudowrinkling— and What to Do About Them

1. *The Sun.* While you're baking on your beach towel, the sun is evaporating the moisture from your skin. Now there's nothing wrong with taking a sunbath, but just be aware of this essential characteristic of sunshine: It dehydrates. The natural dehydrating effect is further enhanced by the swimming that usually accompanies sunbathing. I know this sounds somehow contradictory, but it is a fact that water causes skin dehydration. What else do you think causes the puckers on your fingers after a long swim, bath, or shower?

Not only water itself, but also pool chemicals and the salt in seawater contribute to dehydration. If you like to swim and sun as much as I do, you will take the following precautions. First, use a sunscreen while outdoors. Next, follow up your sunbath with a skin hydrating regimen. As soon as you come in from outdoors, take a cool bath. Lukewarm water may cause less dehydration than hot water. Use an oil of some sort in the bath. Alpha Keri Oil is very good and widely available. Alternately, put a few tablespoons of peanut, olive, Wesson, or baby oil in the bath water and sit in it for five or ten minutes. To hydrate the skin, it must first be immersed in water, then the moisture must be sealed in. The bath oil will help keep in the moisture. When you get out, pat (don't rub) yourself dry and apply a moisturizer that contains urea. You can also seal in your bath's moisture by using a product called Aquaphore or even plain old white Crisco. The trick is to take a small amount and rub it into a large area. Don't worry, you won't smell like a French fry!

If you're sunburned, this regimen will make it considerably less drying and damaging to the skin. If you didn't get a burn, the treatment will help even more by preventing dehydration wrinkles.

Incidentally, smearing baby oil on the skin during a sunbath does absolutely nothing. It doesn't hydrate the skin, since hydration requires prior immersion in water. It in no way enhances the tanning rays, nor does it result in darker tans. What it does best is clog the pores and increase your chance of getting pimples.

2. *Acne Medication.* Some acne treatments have the side effect of causing pseudowrinkles. Why? Because they contain highly effective drying agents that will dehydrate the skin. Sulfur, resorcinol, and alcohol, all frequently contained in acne preparations, are very drying. This is compounded by the high incidence of overapplication of specific products.

So, what should you do if you're taking acne medicines and suddenly noticing wrinkles? First, cut down on the medicine. The strong treatments being prescribed these days must be used gradually. At the start, you shouldn't apply any super medicine more than once a day. Let your tolerance to these products develop a bit, before you totally unleash them on yourself.

When you have stopped medicating your skin, remoisturize it. But if you're acne prone, don't use Crisco, hydrophilic petrolatum, or any oily moisturizer. Use a urea-type product, which chemically attracts and holds moisture without clogging pores. Carmol, which is 20 percent urea, is the strongest. You can also try Cetaphil Lotion, which is a lipid-free (fat-free), non-acnegenic hydrating lotion that you can buy over the counter. Ask your druggist to add a little urea to the Cetaphil, and you'll have a doubly good preparation.

Remember that all soaps tend to be drying, and acne soaps are tremendously drying. For some reason, many acne sufferers tend to develop facial lines and wrinkles because of sunlamp treatments, which are very often a part of the acne therapy. If it's happening to you and you are using a sunlamp, then stop immediately.

3. *Water Pills.* There are basically two groups taking water pills: younger people out to shed pounds of water weight and older folks who take the pills as part of heart disease treatment. Both groups will urinate substantial amounts of water, and the result is often acute dehydration.

When that dehydration causes wrinkles on the face and hands of young people, they can reverse the process simply by stopping the pill and drinking water. Although older people can't stop the pill, lest it jeopardize their heart functions, they can use hydrating creams such as Aquaphore or Crisco again or any oily ointment or moisturizer. Older skin tolerates oil occlusion much better and doesn't tend to get pimples that might otherwise occur. In addition, these oils and ointments will make both the existing pseudowrinkles and age lines look much better.

4. *Winter.* Wintertime dryness, especially the sort that comes from steam-heated houses, is often the cause of pseudowrinkles and dry wrinkling. It happens because your environment is so dry that it dehydrates the skin.

You can guard against this by first cutting down on the number of baths or showers you take. Although showers are less dehydrating than baths, since the skin doesn't become so soaked, you should go easy on both. If you just can't cut down, use Alpha Keri Oil in the bath and keep it short and cool. Then stick with the moisturizers mentioned earlier.

It also helps to buy a humidifier that will spray a fine mist of water into the air. You can get the same effect by lowering the thermostat and putting out tubs of water around your house or apartment. Houseplants will also help moisten a too-dry environment.

Finally, sunlight is often very beneficial to the sort of skin that's prone to wintertime dryness. So get a sunlamp, or take a trip to Florida if you can!

5. *Weight Loss.* Acute, sudden, crazy crash diets don't give the body a chance to fill in areas of loss with collagen, elastin, and the other components of dermal tissue. So the result is temporary wrinkling, which is more acute the older you are.

It's best to lose weight slowly. And if rapid loss is causing you to wrinkle, you can use my magic moisturizer program of warm wet towels and hydrophilic petrolatum (recommended in Chapter 5) or any oily moisturizer. The oily ones work best and cause the greatest cosmetic improvement in the appearance of the wrinkles. But stick to urea-type products if you're prone to acne.

As for permanent wrinkles, there isn't much you can do except cover them with cosmetics or undergo surgery. Or better, leave them uncovered as a badge of wisdom and/or evidence of how long you've been slugging it out with life. The following things cause permanent wrinkles.

1. *Sunshine.* Aside from the pseudowrinkles of sun-induced dehydration, there are the permanent wrinkles of solar elastosis. This term refers to the long-term effect of sun in immoderate doses on unprotected skin. The

cumulative effect of the sun is the destruction of elastic supportive tissue in the dermis. We can actually see how much elastin is gone by doing a biopsy of a small piece of facial skin. The tissue can be stained for elastic material, and if it came from an older tanned and weathered face, nearly all the elastin will appear damaged or degenerated. The medical name for this is basophilic degeneration.

If you've already arrived at that point, you can help matters by reducing the amount of sun you take and wearing a good paba sunscreen when you do sun yourself. The wrinkles and lines on your face might be permanent, but skin hydration will make them look better. Soak the face with a lukewarm wet towel for five minutes, then put on any ointment like hydrophilic petrolatum or even Crisco again. Oily products have a better moisturizing effect than urea products, but they do cause occlusion, which often leads to acne.

Plastic surgery, skin grafts, face-lifts, dermabrasion, and chemical peeling are more radical approaches to (otherwise) permanent wrinkles. These are discussed in Chapter 14.

2. *Smoking.* Several studies have shown that smokers have a high incidence of crow's-feet at the corners of the eyes. No one really knows the reason for this phenomenon, but it has been noted as more prevalent among cigarette smokers than pipe or cigar enthusiasts, and its degree depends on how heavy a smoker you are.

Let's face it, to give up smoking is probably better for you anyway. That web of lines isn't going to go away if you stop, but at least it won't get worse. If you can't or won't quit, you'll find that the oily hydrating ointments mentioned above will help.

3. *Age.* Nothing stops the march of time, and skin progressively deteriorates with advancing age. Wrinkles are an inevitable part of the general loss of water, poor circulation, and deterioration of elastic tissue that comes with the passage of years. It's my feeling that age is more dignified and attractive than most people give it credit for. Whether you feel that way or not, short of surgery, age lines and wrinkles are there to stay. Fortunately, the best oily moisturizers are most effective on older skin.

Chapter 9

Your Skin as an Indicator of Other Disorders

Many common internal disorders show their first symptoms on the skin. And any doctor or internist who does not examine the skin (and hairs and nails too) is simply not giving you a full examination. There are no esoteric conditions described in this chapter, only commonplace human afflictions that are mirrored in the condition of your skin.

Diabetes is a prime example. This is a widespread disease in which the body is incapable of properly absorbing or metabolizing carbohydrates. Usually, the level of unabsorbed sugar in the blood is abnormally high, resulting from a lack of the hormone insulin. Left unattended, diabetes can cause blindness and heart disease.

Diabetic skin manifests several telltale characteristics. Foremost among them is a maddening generalized itch that seems to have no specific cause. When I see scratches and an absence of any skin pathology, diabetes is suspect No. 1. Diabetics are also prone to obesity and a host of surface yeast and fungal infections. A fiery red yeast infection between the fingers with whiteness at the finger crotch is almost always a sign of diabetes. Frequent, recurrent, ferocious boils, itches, abcesses, and fungal infections are a signal that something's wrong. A healthy body gets these things from time to time, but they shouldn't keep recurring. If they do, a good diagnostician will think diabetes.

Two separate skin conditions frequently accompany diabetes. The first goes by the name of diabetic dermopathy and consists of little brown spots that begin to accumulate on the legs and knees. These are caused by poor healing of normal knocks and bumps. In non-diabetics, these small traumas would heal without a trace. Diabetics, however, display particularly poor healing, and these little marks are often—though not always—a tip-off to the existence of the disease. Older people, especially, are prone to diabetic dermopathy, as well as being more susceptible to diabetes in general.

The second skin condition goes by the luxurious name of necrobiosis lipoidica diabeticorum, and if you have it, there's no doubt that you have diabetes as well. It's characterized by an indented, golden yellow lesion that may progress from bad to worse and become ulcerated. Again, you'll usually observe lipoidicas on the legs, and they often have characteristic blood vessels on top.

Liver disease, like diabetes, also shows up on the skin. Your liver is your body's garbage disposal, and when it's diseased or damaged you'll note numerous skin symptoms. The first is jaundice, a yellowing of the skin that is actually rather easy to overlook. When the liver is on the blink, bile salts will accumulate in the bloodstream, causing yellow eyes as well as yellow skin. These salts can also cause itching so severe that it has been known to drive people to suicide. Other typical skin symptoms of liver disease include red palms, thinning of the hair, spider or cherry angiomas (burst blood vessels on the skin surface), even testicular atrophy.

The most common drug used to treat heart ailments is digitalis, and it has its side effects too. Primarily, it tends to cause unnatural breast development in older (fifty-five to sixty) men.

If you've been getting yellowish to white fatty papules around the eyes, it can be an indication of an unhealthy elevated cholesterol level in your bloodstream. These papules are called xanthelasma when they occur around the eyes, and xanthomas when they pop up elsewhere. If you've really been eating rich, what are called eruptive xanthomas can suddenly burst out all over the body after a very fatty meal.

Fortunately, these symptoms can be easily treated by diet, minor surgery in a dermatologist's office, and/or anticholesterol drugs. But their appearance in the first place should be taken as a signal of internal trouble. You would be wise to invest $20 or $30 on a lipid profile of the blood, a test your doctor can administer and assess. It's worth the money to find out the extent of cholesterol in the blood and treat it before irreparable damage is done to the heart.

The skin is also the most obvious indicator of any thyroid disease or imbalance. Thyroid is a common medical problem that can stem not only from a malfunction of the gland itself, but also from undue tension and very frequently from diet pills which contain thyroid. In fact, many thyroid conditions are usually iatrogenic, which means that their cause stems from a doctor's treatment. Either a hyperthyroid person is overtreated to the point that he or she becomes hypothyroid or vice versa!

Hyperthyroid people (with too much thyroid in the blood) look flushed and the skin has a velvety feel.

Hypothyroid (thyroid deficient) people, by contrast, have dry, cracked, coarse, and itchy skin. The complexion tends to be yellowish, and frequently the hair will start to fall out. Despite the dry surface, the skin has a boggy, saturated feel to it, which along with typically enlarged hair follicles is known as the *peau d'orange* (skin of an orange) effect. Hypothyroid imbalances are particularly common among older people. However, sometimes thyroid is prescribed as a pick-me-up for middle-aged people, and the dosage is enough to cause hyperthyroid symptoms. Especially dieters on thyroid-containing diet pills are liable to become hyperthyroid.

The skin is also an excellent way to spot important vitamin imbalances. For example, a deficiency of vitamin C results in poor healing, a tendency to bruise, and abnormally long bleeding. In advanced cases, a lack of this vitamin can show up as little hemorrhages around the hair follicles. It's thought to be impossible to have too much vitamin C.

Too many yellow vegetables with vitamin A, however, causes a yellowing of the skin, particularly on the palms, soles of the feet, and ears. It's called carotenoderma and differs from jaundice in that the whites of the eyes remain unaffected. There are many people who can't metabolize vitamin A well. Even a minimal level, for instance a glass of tomato juice, can turn their ears yellow! However, those with too little vitamin A have another set of symptoms—namely, dry, scaly, mosaic-type skin. The mouth tends to be dry, as do the eyes, which sometimes interferes with vision.

People with sallow lemon-yellow complexions are very often sufferers of pernicious anemia, or lack of vitamin B_{12}. These are often tea and toast folks who eat too lightly and avoid meat and vegetables. The condition is noticeably more common among women with gray hair and blue eyes. The anemic symptoms of B_{12} deficiency don't hit you on the head. Friends might remark that you look "a little pale today," and you might feel somewhat tired. Depending on the extent of the deficiency, your feet might burn, your tongue may become smooth, and vitiligo (whitening of the skin) may set in. A simple blood test will verify the problem and B_{12} injections can solve it.

Some of today's more outlandish diets, so often the topic of fashionable conversation, can be so protein deficient as to play havoc with the skin. Protein in the diet is what keeps fluid in the bloodstream via an osmosis effect. Without sufficient levels, fluid will leak into the skin tissue and make it boggy below, while the surface becomes dry and cracked.

Then there are the farfel-faced people, a marvelously descriptive term for those whose skin is unduly yellow and pale. When the paleness is noted in combination with tremendous itching, it's very often a case of kidney trouble. The itching, incidentally, is thought to be caused by a buildup of by-products in the skin that would otherwise be eliminated by a normally functioning kidney.

In the case of cancer, it is generally true that you will have discovered it before the symptoms reach the skin. However, certain signs of internal cancer have made their way into dermatological literature. Generalized and persistent itching without apparent cause is one of these signs. So is the sudden appearance of a beard of soft hair on a woman. Called hypertrichosis langunosa, this onset of unexpected facial hair is often associated with cancer. In men, a similarly sudden onset of female secondary sex characteristics (such as enlarged breasts) is a danger signal too.

Cancer can also cause what are called acanthosis nigricans. These are black thickenings of the skin, velvety to the touch, and look like little church spires. Most frequently they occur in the underarms and sometimes on the tongue, and they usually signal some kind of internal malignancy in the gastrointestinal tract. However, occasionally fat people will have what look to be the same thing, even though there is no cancer present. When this is true, the condition is called pseudo-acanthosis nigricans.

The appearance of a forest of localized seborrheic keratoses (itchy, warty, dark brown, greasy lesions, mentioned in Chapter 11) is known as a sign of Lesser and Trelat. Sometimes it means there is a cancer in an organ directly below.

I would say that one of the most typical reasons for a visit to a dermatologist is persistent itching with no specific rash. The patients will describe it to me, even though there is no obvious sign of anything wrong on the skin. Most times, the itch is due to nothing but dryness, and it's easily reversible by hydration. But by now you can see that there are often many other and more serious causes. If you suffer from unrelenting itching, it certainly behooves you to get three simple tests: a CBC (complete blood count), a blood sugar test (for diabetes), and a sedimentation test (which can reveal a host of internal problems that are keyed to the rate red blood cells settle out of the clear plasma).

Anyone who pays normal attention to his or her skin should be able to note the following and take appropriate action. If you're too yellow, it can be a sign of kidney disease, vitamin B_{12} deficiency, and sometimes an excess of vitamin A. Unduly pale complexions can mean any anemia, an iron deficiency, or any source of internal bleeding (ulcer, hemorrhoid, cancer). And if you're too ruddy, it can be a case of hyperthyroid or what's called secondary polycythemia. In this latter condition, the lungs are diseased to the point where not enough oxygen is getting into the blood. The body then produces extra red cells and the result is a flushed red skin. If your skin is red and you are sluggish, you may have a condition known as the Pickwickian syndrome. Named after the Dickens character, this syndrome probably brings three or four people each day into every major hospital.

Chapter 10

What's Catching and What Isn't

Fortunately, most common skin diseases are not contagious. Furthermore, there are degrees of contagion. Some things are definitely catching—if you touch it, you get it. But most others are either mildly catching or not catching at all. By mildly catching, I mean that it is possible to pick up the disease if you literally rub your nose in it for a long enough period of time. If it's not catching, that means you can touch it fearlessly.

What's Not Catching?

As I say, most things aren't. Here's a list of a dozen of the most common skin diseases, none of which is catching at all, and each of which is usually (and incorrectly) suspected of being highly contagious.

eczema
poison ivy
skin cancer
acne

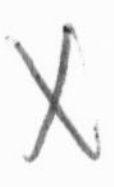

psoriasis
dandruff
shingles
skin tumors
sweat retention syndrome
lichen planus
alopecia areata
pityriasis rosea

Probably 90 percent of the people who just read this list are not really sure they believe it. Doesn't poison ivy spread among children like wildfire? No it doesn't. Children often play together in the same patch, however, and the simultaneous exposure often gives the illusion of a contagious spread. How about eczema and psoriasis, you might ask; don't they often plague a whole family? Yes they do, but it's a genetic predisposition that makes a person prone to these conditions in the first place.

If someone has alopecia areata (the moth-eaten balding discussed in Chapter 4), you can use his or her comb with safety. And if a good friend suffers from the explosive body-wide eruptions of pityriasis rosea, go ahead and shake his hand. It's OK!

But having said that, I must now point out that if you suffer from any of these diseases, you yourself can easily make them or any other condition highly contagious. How do you do it? By scratching the lesions and causing a secondary bacterial infection. Infections of this sort are called impetigo. Impetigo always manifests the same highly characteristic symptom whether you started out with poison ivy or psoriasis. The symptom is golden yellow crusts that form over a superficial oozing. And though the original disease might not have been catching, once it is impetiginized it becomes very contagious. The bacteria that commonly result in impetigo are staph and strep, but oral penicillin treatment will curb them quickly and effectively.

What's Mildly Catching?

Of course, what's mildly catching for the average person can be much more so for certain individuals. It's a matter of end organ sensitivity.

Viral diseases are a good case in point. Most people don't get them from contact, but there are a few who do. The most common viral skin disease is warts. The wart virus proliferates in the skin and produces benign tumors, usually flesh-colored but occasionally whitish or yellowish. You can get warts as easily on the face as on the fingers, and as easily on the genitals as the toes. Although traditionally associated with younger people, more and more older patients with wart complaints are visiting my office. The virus likes warmth and moisture and warts often locate on children's fingers and mouths, on the faces of young adults (particularly the beard area on young men), on the genitals of either sex, and frequently on the anus area of homosexuals.

The plantar wart—incorrectly suspected as the scourge of the antebellum South—is so-called because it appears on the plantar surface of the tarsus bone, otherwise known as the bottom of your foot. And where there's one plantar wart, there's usually another nearby or on the way. Are they catching? I've probably taken off thousands of warts in my practice, and I've only "caught" one in my life. Even so, it's not a foregone conclusion that I picked up the virus from exposure.

The wart virus additionally has a long incubation period, possibly as long as three months. So it's very difficult to tell when or how you picked it up. But once you've got it, you are very contagious to yourself! A common syndrome that plagues many young men results from scraping a wart while shaving—soon hundreds of little warts appear all over the face.

Warts are eccentric and everybody reacts differently, both to the warts and to the methods of removal. Every doctor has a few wart stories, and I will share with you the experience of my own wart. At first it seemed as if nothing would get rid of it. I burned it off with an electric needle—it came back. Then I froze it off with liquid nitrogen, and it came back again. Finally, I began to shave it down every day with a razor and it went away.

In most cases, however, either the electric needle or the liquid nitrogen application is plenty. And sometimes the doctor can apply cauterizing chemicals to the area and kill the virus. You yourself can remove warts from your feet if you have the ability to scrape off dead skin. Go out and buy a 40 percent salicylic acid plaster from a druggist, cut out a size slightly larger than necessary, apply it to the wart, and leave it on for a week. During that time, the skin under the plaster will become white and deadened. At the end of the week, scrape and slice away the dead tissue and continue to apply new plasters until the remainder of the wart has been removed. Typically, this process will last from four to six weeks, but naturally that's not everybody's timetable.

When warts invade the rectal or genital areas, they present particularly difficult problems. It's so warm and moist there that the wart virus thrives in defiance of many treatments. Often your doctor will apply podophyllyn, an organic antiviral medicine that's pretty effective even though it burns like crazy. The usual treatment is for the doctor to apply it at his office, then have the patient wash it off four to six hours later at home. The patient then returns to the doctor for renewed applications every three or four weeks until the wart is gone.

Another example of a common disease widely thought to be very contagious is molluscum contagiosum—even the name would surely seem to indicate that it's catching. Caused by the largest virus that infects man, and characterized by multiple grouped yellowish papules with a central concave dell, its usual victim is a child. Before you know it he's covered with them. They spread with speed on one person, but hardly ever spread from one person to another.

While you must totally destroy a wart, a molluscum is much easier to kill. The virus is big but tender, and the doctor need only destroy the environment of the lesion to kill it. He can do this simply by nicking off the top of each papule. They don't even bleed much and this simple operation is practically foolproof. The only danger is that the doctor will miss one little papule. If that happens, they'll reappear in force equal to the original occurrence. But get every single one, and they won't come back.

If you're not a young parent struggling with an outbreak of molluscum, you might be a young single (or married for that matter) struggling with herpes simplex. The name again is less than descriptive, since herpes is anything but simplex. The hallmark of herpes is that it hurts. It's caused by a pair of related viruses and its reputation for contagiousness is under much medical scrutiny.

Herpes type 1 almost always occurs above the waist; type 2 occurs with similar consistency below the waist. The two viruses are in the same family and are in fact indistinguishable without the aid of an electron microscope. They produce the same lesions but in different spots. These lesions consist of multiple groups of little blisters on an inflamed base, and they're very tender. Type 1 is usually on the lips, and we call it a cold sore or fever blister more often than we call it herpes. Type 2 appears on the penis or the vagina, where it is usually recognized as herpes right away. The pain is what makes it so distinctive.

How does one get herpes? No one knows for sure. How it does get into the system is a mystery, but once it's there, it seems to just wait for the inevitable traumas that come in the course of everybody's life. Fever, stress, tiredness, illness, or even simple sun exposure can set off a type 1 reaction. Type 2 can arise from any of these plus sex, physical trauma, heat, or other infections.

Having sex with someone who has herpes is sometimes followed by an appearance of the lesions on yourself. But this does not mean you picked up the virus by contact. Remember, the human body hosts a tremendous variety of organisms, and there's nothing strange about herpes being one of them.

The most widely practiced treatment is to do nothing at all. Herpes comes, hurts, then usually goes away all by itself. Some people get it more than once, however, and want to do something about it. The best home remedy is the application of a little alcohol to help dry the lesions up, plus a topical anesthetic for the pain. Any of the "-caine" preparations will do fine, like Solarcaine, which is normally used for sunburn but works well here. Caladryl and some of the other poison ivy medications are good too. If it really hurts, have your doctor prescribe Xylocaine ointment, so you can wait out the virus in more comfort; however, be careful. Many of the "-caine" preparations are allergenic.

If you're treating yourself, you might want to try a little antibacterial cream to avoid infection. Bacitracin is a good OTC preparation that's widely available. Whatever you do, don't use any steroid creams. They may reduce inflammation in other conditions, but they'll spread a virus infection. And take heart—herpes is very rarely a serious problem.

Nonetheless, some people have recurrent episodes that become such a problem they are driven to find a cure. This is sad, since no good therapy is really available. At this writing, there is a vaccine that has been formulated in Europe, but it's so new as to be yet unnamed. Effectiveness is about 70 percent to 80 percent, but the question is largely academic since the FDA has not yet approved it for use in the United States. I have a patient who has herpes eruptions literally every time she has sex. She's going to Germany to undergo the vaccine. But if you can't afford Germany, you'll have to make do with either symptomatic treatments like alcohol and Solarcaine or resort to a very limited mixed bag of more stringent modalities.

For example, you probably have had a smallpox vaccination at some point in your life, and you'll remember that the vaccine was smeared onto a scratch the doctor made on your arm. There is a theory held by some that multiple small injections of smallpox vaccine (as opposed to being smeared on a scratch) will have the effect of stimulating your system to produce more antibodies. These antibodies are then supposed to kill the herpes virus, which is rather similar to the smallpox virus. There is certainly logic to the observation that people with continual herpes episodes probably don't have good antibodies. Therefore, this treatment might be worth a try.

Some doctors try to kill the virus by photo-inactivation. This plan requires the lesions to be painted with a dye that clings to the virus. When light is shown on a virus with dye attached, it will die. These dyes are available by prescription, but they don't always work. Furthermore, there is an inherent danger in trying to effect a change of this sort in the body. It's unpredictable, and the cure might possibly be worse than the disease. How? Well, the virus could, for example, be transformed into a cancer-causing virus. This risk is slim but does exist.

This chapter has so far specialized in misleadingly named diseases, and it's not over yet. Athlete's foot is next, but athletes are not the prime sufferers. In fact, the disease most frequently—although not exclusively—afflicts diabetics and fat people! It's a fungal infection of the superficial skin of the foot. The symptoms include whiteness and moisture between the fourth and fifth toe and fissuring (cracking) between the toes. If left unattended the symptoms can escalate to include thickening of the sole (which becomes red and scaly) and contagion of the nails. When athlete's foot hits the nails, the problem can become almost insoluble. But until that point, it's effectively treated by any of the numerous OTC athlete's foot preparations, many of which are very widely advertised. Of all the products available, I recommend Tinactin, which comes in either liquid, cream, or powder form. The liquid is perhaps the easiest to use, and the powder does nicely as a prophylactic dust for shoes and socks.

Let me state again that it is really hard to pick up athlete's foot by exposure. In fact, you can literally bathe cut feet in the fungi without catching it. Who gets it, then? You have to be susceptible to catch it. It seems to afflict a certain body mold, not the athletic type either. People who are susceptible to fungal infections, such as the diabetics mentioned above, will catch it without ever being in a locker room, just because they are prone to coming down with fungus infections. Healthy athletes can slog through the fungus every day on the way to the shower and never have a problem.

The Most Catching Skin Diseases

After all this talk about diseases that are not contagious, it's time to warn you about what *is*. And I wish to preface this discussion by noting that once you begin therapy for any of the below, you generally stop being contagious. This is not a matter of becoming a leper.

First on the list is syphilis, and I refer you to Chapter 12 for a detailed description of why this particular venereal disease is a skin disease and what you can do about it.

The second most common catching skin disease in adults is scabies. This is an infestation of little burrowing mites that dig into your skin. They cause multiple, grouped, itchy papules, frequently near the waist and/or wrist areas and between the fingers. They can also appear on the genitals even though they are not specifically a venereal disease. They are enormously contagious, and the treatment for the sufferer (and for her or his friends too) is a marvelously named medication called Kwell.

Ringworm infections of the scalp are also very contagious. The symptoms are scaly red balding patches on the head, but this should not be confused with alopecia areata, whose bald patches are neither inflamed nor catching. Ringworm very often shows up first on children who play with the family dog. Before you know it, the whole family is breaking out. The treatment is usually pills or a topical medicine for the whole family and the dog too. The pills normally prescribed are called griseofulvin, and they work well enough, despite certain side effects. Griseofulvin seems to cause headaches, is photosensitizing, causes allergic reactions in people who are also allergic to penicillin, and is quite expensive. Hopefully, a sturdy topical modality such as Tinactin will be enough for you.

Chapter 11

Skin Cancer: Yes or No?

Most cases of skin cancer do not spread readily to other organs, can often be treated without surgery, and getting it does not necessarily mean that you are cancer-prone. In fact, often skin cancer is cancer in name only and most people overreact to it. This is not to say that cancer is not dangerous. It is, and there's an epidemic of it raging across this country today. But skin cancer is a special breed, and, with rare exceptions, it's not nearly as dangerous as people think.

Many frightening things aren't cancer in the first place. Human skin, especially older skin with long years of accumulated sun exposure, is capable of manifesting a wild assortment of lesions. I would say that nine out of every ten patients who come to my office thinking they have cancer in fact do not have it at all. Most lumps and bumps, even those that alarmingly change color and size, are quite benign and are associated only with advancing age. This fact should comfort you, but by all means don't rely on self-diagnosis. Only your doctor can tell you for sure what it is you have.

Seven Not-So-Deadly Lumps and Bumps

The following common conditions may seem terrifying at first, but each and every one is quite benign. They are not cancers, despite some flamboyant symptoms.

Seborrheic Keratoses. These lesions occur mainly on the trunk, but they can also appear on the face or scalp. Classically, you'll see them on the bodies of old women at the beach. They are raised and warty-looking and appear to be stuck onto the skin's surface. In fact, it's quite easy to scrape them off with a fingernail. The color ranges from brown to murky yellow, and it's possible to observe little blackheads within the lesion.

Seborrheic keratoses are cosmetically ugly but quite harmless. They do tend to grow, especially in areas irritated by belts or bras that knock them off. Some patients witness a scary proliferation of them—but the disease is quite benign and not cancerous. When scraped off, nine times out of ten they won't reoccur. They're so harmless that unless they bother you, leave them alone.

Skin Tags. The medical name for a skin tag is papilloma, and the medical cause is simply unknown. These are little outpatchings of skin typically under the arms, on the sides of the neck, and on the cheeks. They come in groups and can be frightening.

Although the cause is unknown, skin tags just never turn into cancer. In my opinion, most of them should be left alone. The patient who feels they're too disfiguring can have his or her doctor cut or burn them off. Specific modalities for removal of these conditions are discussed a little later in this chapter. Removal is not a major undertaking, and your doctor can do many at one sitting.

Syringomas. These papules appear in groups, and they mainly plague women. They appear symmetrically under the eyes or flanking the nose.

A syringoma is really a benign tumor caused by an enlargement of a sweat duct. To remove them is quite easy, but there is a particular danger of scarring. Under-eye tissue is very delicate, so I usually advise that you leave them alone if possible. Again, they pose no threat to overall health.

Histiocytomas. Usually solitary and well-rounded, these firm little nodules (bigger than a papule) are common. They are often located on the extremities—near the knees, elbows, hips—and are thought to be a body response to some (often repeated) trauma.

The dermis layer of the skin contains special cells called histiocytes. These cells help repair the skin after a trauma by aiding in the production of collagen and fibrosis. A histiocytoma, however, is a case of bodily overreaction. Too much fibrous tissue has been created, resulting in a tough, raised lesion. What's worse, the doctor must further traumatize the lesion in order to biopsy it, which sometimes aggravates and enlarges what you've got already. Not too attractive perhaps, but these lesions are not cancerous.

Senile Lentigo. These are the classic "liver spots" you see on the hands and faces of older people. They can occasionally turn into skin cancer, but the conversion is extremely rare. The vast majority are quite benign.

The senile lentigo lesion is not raised, which makes it especially hard to eradicate. Trichloroacetic acid or various other caustic agents will burn it off, as will electric needles. It's probably better just to leave it alone.

Sebaceous Hyperplasia. You might really call this "aged acne." The lesions measure a half inch across and are shiny, yellow, waxy-oily tumors. They're located on the face, especially the nose, and although they are quite benign, they do bear a resemblance to certain cancers. Be sure to get a doctor's diagnosis.

I call this particular bump "aged acne" because it is a benign enlargement of an oil gland. If you're courageous, open it with a pin, and express (squeeze out) some of the fat inside. Or your doctor can remove it with methods described later in this chapter. Ironically, it's a good sign if a lot of them develop at once. The cancers they so closely resemble do not appear in groups.

Actinic Keratoses. The papules that distinguish this condition are slightly raised, red, scaly, and usually (though not always) come in groups. They appear typically on sun-exposed areas and when biopsied show evidence of slight disorganization. Most doctors feel that actinic keratoses are *almost* a cancer—or at least precancerous—and should be removed. Topical 5-fluorouracil is particularly effective, as is cryosurgery (freezing the lesions with liquid nitrogen, then scraping them off). The latter method is preferable when there are lots of lesions.

Modalities for Removing Things (Cancerous or Otherwise)

I'm hoping in this chapter to allay a lot of widely held fears about skin cancer. But I don't want to replace them with complacency. When you get a bump, *always* have a biopsy. It's common practice in most places for independent laboratories, and not the doctor himself, to conduct biopsy tests.

Many of the lesions mentioned above are removed simply by scraping the skin with either a scalpel blade or an instrument called a curette. This latter looks like a comedone extractor; it's a stainless steel hand tool with a small bottomless cup at the end. The open bottom has sharp edges, which pry away a raised lesion. If the lesion isn't raised already, an injection of Xylocaine into the skin will raise it.

Sometimes an electric needle is used. The doctor holds a stylus whose point emits raw cutting electricity. The amount of juice is regulated on a control box and with a foot pedal.

There are a number of chemical approaches too. Trichloroacetic acid is a favorite modality because of its caustic properties. It also precipitates out when in contact with certain skin proteins. This characteristic acts as a built-in safety valve, stopping the caustic effect before it does too much. Some doctors have occasion to use liquid nitrogen, which freezes a lesion off. And, of course, there's the previously mentioned topical 5-fluorouracil, which is used to destroy disorganized tissue.

DNCB (dinitrochlorobenzene) is a new and experimental modality that destroys tissue through allergic reaction. DNCB is remarkable stuff for the reason that almost anybody can be sensitized to it. Remember that allergic reactions can only happen in people who are sensitized to (and whose bloodstreams have produced antibodies against) an allergen. If you don't have an allergic reaction, it's either because you've never been exposed or because there's nothing in the substance that provokes your bloodstream into antibody production.

Not so with DNCB. You can paint it on anybody, and their body will develop strong antibodies. So strong, that the next time DNCB touches the skin, or specifically one of the lesions mentioned above, a terrific local allergic reaction can effectively destroy lesion and tissue alike. When the response runs its course, healthy tissue grows back.

The last major modality is the X ray, and I've saved it for last since it's primarily used against cancer. This brings us to the real thing, and how to recognize it.

Three Types of Skin Cancer

Basal Cell Carcinoma. This is the least malignant and most common form of skin cancer. It consists of shiny, pearly nodules, with characteristic blood vessels visible on top. It may or may not be ulcerated (have a hole in the middle), and it most commonly occurs on sun-exposed areas of the skin. It can, however, turn up anywhere.

Basal cell is a frequent complaint of fair-skinned people living in very sunny climates. There's a lot of it in Australia and in Arizona. It varies from the size of a button to covering an entire face. It kills skin locally but does not pollute the bloodstream. So the treatment is to cut it off; and even if it reoccurs, it can be re-excised or X-rayed. In point of fact, under proper supervision, 99 percent of patients recover completely.

I see perhaps two or three people every day with this complaint. They've had it, on an average, for some six months before they sought professional help. The treatment is desiccation (drying up) with the electric needle and curettage (scooping out) with the curette until the cancerous tissue is cut out completely. X rays are effective too, but their drawback is a tendency to make the skin look bad in twenty years. They're a better treatment for a seventy-year-old man than for a thirty-year-old woman.

Squamous Cell Carcinoma. Squamous is a little worse than basal, but it's still not too malignant. Again, it usually does not pollute the bloodstream, although it can, and it responds well to surgery or chemicals. It simply requires more vigorous treatment.

The lesions themselves look distinctively different. They are not shiny, but instead are scaly red papules without blood vessels on top. Sometimes they're ulcerated and sometimes they're not. The specific treatment depends on the age and location of the lesions.

Malignant Melanoma. This is the worst sort of skin cancer, but fortunately it's very rare. People with malignant melanoma have a very poor prognosis.

The cancer is thought to arise from cells that produce melanin, the protein coloring agent. It usually evidences itself as a spreading brown to black patch, but there are many other possible colors. The rate of spread is just as variable. Melanoma is often very hard to diagnose. It can start anywhere there's pigment, even in the eye. Ironically, it's rare in black people.

The treatment consists of wide excision or chemotherapy, but substantive discussion is beyond the scope of this book.

What to Do If You Have a Skin Lesion

Have a spot, a lump, or a bump? Well, chances are it's nothing serious, so first relax. Next, ask your doctor if a biopsy is necessary—and trust him if he says no. Even if the lesion is horrifying you with color changes and/or bleeding, it may not be as serious as you think. And all sorts of tried and true treatments are available.

However, some treatments are more advisable than others. If you're worried about cosmetic damage to your appearance, tell your doctor. Surgery, for instance, is less damaging than desiccation (with the electric needle). And X rays, as mentioned earlier, heal well initially but turn up as very unattractive marks after a passage of many years. Just remember that your doctor has plenty of latitude to tailor a treatment for you.

Chapter 12

VD and Its Effects on the Skin

Dermatologists have historically been associated with the treatment of syphilis. It was the successful prepenicillin treatment of the disease with heavy metals in the nineteenth century that marked the beginning of dermatology as a modern specialty.

The connection is a natural one. Skin rashes—syphilitic and otherwise—have understandably always been taken to skin doctors. Even today, most doctors will refer a VD patient immediately to a dermatologist. And it is also true that many people with rashes or bumps on the genitals will go to a dermatologist in a big city rather than to their family doctor in their local town.

Before I launch into the subject of syphilis, I would like to note here that most sores on the penis or vagina are not syphilitic. These sores bring millions into dermatology offices every year, but syphilis actually is not very common; most sores on the genitals stem from other causes.

Worse Things Could Happen to You Than Syphilis

Tertiary syphilis is the end of the road for people who have it, but comparatively few cases ever come to this point. This disease is surrounded with deadly myths, and I intend to expose as many as possible.

To begin with, you can only catch it if you're exposed to the organism itself. This typically happens through contact with an open syphilitic sore. Syphilis carriers don't exude a poisonous air of contagion, and unless you're unlucky enough to touch an open lesion, it is difficult to be infected. The organism itself happens to be rather delicate and only survives in nearly ideal (warm and wet) conditions. Toilet seats or towels won't infect you since the organism can't survive on them.

The disease goes through three progressive stages, called respectively primary, secondary, and tertiary syphilis. Infection requires moist-area contact with another moist area, which is why sex provides such ideal circumstances. Four to six weeks after exposure to the bacteria, the characteristic sore of primary syphilis makes its debut. It occurs wherever the organism touched you—on the penis, scrotum, anus, labia, perhaps within the vagina. Female interior plumbing, as it happens, makes diagnosis in women particularly difficult. For although the sore is obvious, it is quite painless. If it's hidden within the vagina, the woman might never know she had it.

I don't advise it, but it's quite possible to have sex with a syphilitic person and not become infected. You may just be lucky enough to avoid the open sore, or the sore may have already healed on the carrier and rendered him or her non-contagious. The sore itself is easy to identify once spotted. It is hard and usually ulcerated (has a hole in the middle). The absence of tenderness is a good diagnostic indication of syphilis.

Primary syphilis presents several unique pitfalls for the sufferer. The biggest one stems from the fact that if left untreated, the sore will go away all by itself in two to three weeks. This leads countless sufferers to ignore and/or forget all about the sore ever happening.

It is also possible to get the sore, go for a blood test, and have a negative result. Too many people wrongly assume that blood tests never lie, without understanding how the blood tests work. The most popular one is called the VDRL, and owes its name to an organization called the Venereal Disease Research Lab. But this test does not indicate the presence of the syphilis bacteria. What it tests for is the presence of a syphilis antibody, which your bloodstream produces to combat the bacteria. Therefore, a problem sometimes arises when a VDRL test is given to a recently infected person whose body has not yet had time to manufacture the necessary antibodies. Result: negative test, even though syphilis is indeed present.

To avoid this, people who have had a negative VDRL are advised to wait six to eight weeks and have another VDRL. The time elapsed allows the body further opportunity to produce the telltale antibodies.

There is another test to verify the presence of syphilis; it's called a dark-field examination. This consists of taking a sample of ooze from the sore and examining it under a dark-field microscope. This instrument illuminates the specimen from the side and actually shows it up quite clearly. The syphilis bacteria is a distinctively corkscrew-like organism called a spirochete. If it's present in the sample, it's easy to spot swimming around under the microscope. However, often the sores have been swabbed with iodine or washed with antibacterial soap. This will kill the spirochetes on the surface, result in a negative dark-field reading, but leave the spirochetes alive and well below the skin's surface.

Some people think they can take penicillin orally and not get syphilis. Don't try it. Penicillin works remarkably well against the spirochete, but it's practically impossible to get an effective blood level of penicillin short of an injection. This is true in general of antibiotics. They don't make good prophylactics since too high a blood level is needed for them to work. What's worse, popping a few penicillin pills can actually mask the effects of primary syphilis and disguise the fact that you've got it. It distorts blood test results too.

At this point, I wish to inject (if you'll pardon the expression) that other things besides penicillin work effectively on the syphilis spirochete. If you're allergic to penicillin, your doctor can recommend erythromycin or tetracycline to avoid sometimes dangerous allergic reactions.

Of course, if you do nothing at all, the sore will go away, but new symptoms will emerge about six weeks later in the form of a distinctive rash. At this point it's called secondary syphilis and is comprised of ham-colored, non-itchy, slightly scaly, bumpy, oval-shaped patches that are quite widespread all over the body. The rash particularly shows up on the palms and the soles of the feet, two places where rashes very rarely occur under normal circumstances. By now the patient will usually go to a doctor if he didn't when the initial lesion arose. The VDRL is almost always positive in the secondary phase, and the spirochete can be effectively treated with about two to four times as much penicillin as would have been required during the first stage.

Still, there are pitfalls here too. Most normal people would go to a doctor with a rash like this, but there are some who won't. And if they don't, the rash goes away in two weeks all by itself. This phenomenon can again postpone a visit to the doctor. But then comes a period of usually a month or two in which the rash comes back, then goes away, comes back, goes away, and so on, and so on. It can seesaw like this for a few months whether you treat it or not.

When you do treat it, the rash tends to "light up," as we say. This means the lesions become bigger and redder, while you can get very sick to your stomach.

Without treatment, a patient will move from secondary syphilis into what's called latent syphilis. In the latent period, you'll have positive blood tests but no symptoms. In fact, this phase can last forever and many syphilitics can and do finish life without any major symptoms and without ever infecting anybody. This without ever having had any treatment!

But whereas the statistical odds may be in the favor of the man or woman who has never had treatment, the threat of tertiary syphilis will loom until death. This is an awful prospect, and the person who is aware of the infection but doesn't get treatment is simply stupid. What kicks latent into the tertiary phase? Probably just bad luck. When it happens, the spirochetes can do all sorts of horrible damage. The brain, spinal cord, and nervous system can be invaded, resulting in disintegration of those systems together with insanity. Major blood vessels can burst; the nose cartilage can degenerate; you can go blind; the list is long and devastating.

Tertiary syphilis mainly shows up on people who live in closets. Society tests us over and over, and it's difficult to arrive at the tertiary level today. When we have babies, when we get married or go into the army, we always have blood tests. So aware is government of the progress of syphilis that it even prescribes specific treatment levels of penicillin.

I mentioned earlier that the VDRL can give a negative reading even when you've got syphilis, because your body hasn't had time to manufacture necessary antibodies. The test can trip up for another reason too, called the prozone phenomenon. This happens when the blood is supersaturated with the spirochete and the accompanying antibody. Under these conditions, the VDRL reads negative. When I see obvious secondary symptoms and a negative test, I immediately suspect the prozone phenomenon. The antibodies just physically refuse to conform to the test; why it happens isn't understood. However, if the blood is diluted and tested again, the results will properly indicate syphilis.

It is also possible to have a biologically false positive response to the VDRL. This is because it is a nonspecific test that will indicate the presence of other things besides syphilis antibodies. Among these other things are hepatitis, mononucleosis, leprosy, the common cold (true!), and a selection of extremely rare diseases. On these occasions, however, it's usually a very weak positive test.

It's possible to check up on your VDRL, and this is automatically done in many places. There's a very specific test for syphilis, and the only reason it hasn't supplanted the VDRL is because it takes much longer and costs a great deal more. It's called the fluorescent treponemal antibody test (FTA), and the results leave little doubt.

If you've ever had syphilis, good advice for you would be to have a VDRL every year. It may well surprise you to discover a positive reading for syphilis when you thought you were cured. Even if your case was adequately treated, antibodies may linger in the bloodstream long after the spirochete is gone.

So, how do you tell if you've contracted a new case? Simply by noting if your regularly positive VDRL is unusually vehement. You can expect some variability in each year's test, but a big jump means either a new case or reactivation of an old one.

There's an Epidemic of Gonorrhea

Actually, gonorrhea has hardly any skin manifestations. It's mentioned here mainly because in the minds of most people it occupies a place directly next to syphilis. And, whereas syphilis is not common, gonorrhea has reached epidemic proportions.

The major symptom is a yellow to green, sloppy-looking pus discharged during often painful attempts to urinate. You could call it diarrhea of the penis or vagina. If left untreated—and it's particularly hard to diagnose in women, because of their interior structure—the bacteria can invade the bloodstream and result in pustular, red-based lesions on the extremities. If it comes to this point, you've really neglected it. At its worst, gonorrhea can destroy the reproductive system.

Treatment is easy and usually consists of penicillin or oral tetracycline.

Herpes

Whereas women usually come to my office for acne, probably half the men I see come in with a sore on the penis. The sore in most instances is the result of a fairly innocent trauma of some kind—an abrasion, a cut, a bite, a zipper accident. These lesions are typically elongated, fairly painful, and go away nicely with only a few dabs of zinc oxide or Bacitracin ointment.

But sometimes the lesion is caused by the herpes virus. In that case, it consists of grouped, painful little blisters that often appear on the genitals after mental traumas, as well as after a physical graze or abrasion. Left alone, they usually just run their course and disappear. When they don't, an elaborate treatment is required, details of which are included in Chapter 10.

The above description pertains to what's called type 2 herpes. Type 1 herpes is caused by a different but closely related virus. The major symptom of type 1 is the familiar ulcerated cold sore that has landed on nearly everyone's lip at one time or another. These two viruses are picked up separately, but it is unclear whether the virus waits in your system for a trauma or whether the trauma itself is the occasion of the introduction of the virus into your system. In any case, it is interesting to note that stress seems to trigger type 1 as often as type 2.

Primary Irritant Dermatitis of the Penis/Vagina

The warm and moist environment of the genitals is the ideal place for any irritant to fester. Sometimes what looks like VD is only a case of skin irritation, especially where there's redness and small ulcerations.

Substances that most commonly irritate the genital tissue include urine, female hygiene sprays, contraceptive jellies and foams, dried semen, lubricating preparations on some condoms, and unusually harsh douches. This might be the simple explanation to your problem, in which case you can breathe a big sigh of relief, start keeping the genital area extra clean, and have your doctor prescribe a mild cream.

Scabies

This is a very itchy eruption of grouped papules that can occur anywhere on the body but frequently is seen on the waistline and buttocks. It is caused by an infestation of mites that crawl under the skin and lay eggs. Scabies incidence has reached epidemic proportions, and it's very contagious not only from sexual activity but from mere close proximity. This is the venereal disease that you can catch from sitting on an infected toilet seat.

People scratch these eruptions like crazy, causing the doctor to miss the diagnosis completely. A good clue is the presence of the rash between the fingers, as scabies is one of the very few conditions to show up there. But it's often too tempting to prescribe a steroid cream for the itching and forget about the bug that's causing it!

Effective treatment consists of total body application of Kwell. You keep it on anywhere from four to twenty-four hours, depending on your doctor and your condition. This treatment is repeated three times: today, tomorrow, and a week from tomorrow. Kwell works extremely well.

Crabs

Just as scabies are only mites, crabs are only lice. There are many kinds of lice, and they infest different parts of the clothing and body. Pubic lice only live in the warm, moist environment of the genitals, where they can itch like crazy. They look like tiny white specks that move around.

The treatment is the same as for scabies—total body immersion in Kwell. It's a good idea to have your bed partner similarly treated, since crabs are usually contracted during sex.

While these conditions are the most common in the United States, the rest of the world is suffering from a wild (from our standpoint) array of venereal esoterica. In the Far East, for instance, many people fall prey to chancroid, which is a disease characterized by extremely painful and ragged ulcerations on the genitals. But in the States, this condition is rare. In our part of the world, most cases of VD will fall into one of the above categories.

Chapter 13

Medication and Your Skin

Consider the average American's daily intake of foreign substances. Mouthwash, aspirin, toothpaste, deodorant soap, stomach antacids, artificial sweeteners, chemical ingredients, all contribute to an indisputable conclusion: We are overmedicated. The people who take upwards of a dozen prescription pills a day really dramatize this situation—it's amazing they don't rattle!

Even those of us who aren't pill poppers would probably be better off with fewer of these artificial ingredients inside us. The reason for this is the steady and almost inevitable process of sensitization that occurs within the body. Eventually, sensitization leads to allergic reaction. It may take a week, or maybe twenty years, or maybe you'll discontinue the medication before you become sensitized. But statistically, a high intake of many different medications leads to an inevitably greater risk of becoming sensitized to one or more of them.

As far as your skin is concerned, sensitization can result in what's called a drug eruption. The first part of this chapter itemizes a baker's dozen of the most frequently observed eruptions. Following that is a short list of commonly used medications that can sometimes cause skin problems.

Remember that whether or not you react to any of these substances is an individual matter. Many people glide through life without so much as a rash. However, increasing numbers of people do suffer from drug-induced eruptions. And the more pills and medicines we consume as a nation, the greater the problem becomes. Please note that for simplicity's sake I've sometimes used trade names instead of complicated chemical names.

Thirteen Unlucky Drug Eruptions

1. *Exanthems.* Exanthematic people are suffering from a generalized, symmetrically balanced rash on the body. It has a very specific brick-red color, so specific in fact that dermatologists refer to the color as "drug-red." Along with the rash, some patients suffer from fever, others get lesions inside the mouth, and still others have an overall sick feeling. And while some sufferers experience all of these additional symptoms, others suffer from only the rash and otherwise feel fine.

Drug-red eruptions occur when a person has taken enough of a certain medicine to become sensitized. And again, we all have different thresholds of reactivity, so the allergic reaction is not predictable. Commonly taken medications associated with the drug-red response after sensitization include:

penicillin
aspirin
water pills
barbiturates
tetracyclines (used in acne treatments)

gold (widely used for arthritis)
Dilantin (used as a treatment for convulsions)
vaccination serums (you can become allergic to any serum—from snakebite to polio)

2. *Hives.* These are the familiar raised bumps that almost all of us have had at one time or another. The wheal (bump) itself is white and surrounded by red, inflamed-looking skin. Here's something to remember: Aspirin not only can cause hives, it tends to make them worse whether or not it's the original cause. The following medications will sometimes cause a hive reaction:

aspirin
penicillin
Ampicillin (a popular antibiotic)
Dilantin
Darvon
birth-control pills
codeine
water pills
penicillin (at the injection site)
insulin (at the injection site)

3. *Photoallergic Eruptions.* Although these bumps require the presence of sunlight, as well as the causative drug, no excessive dose of desert-strength sun is needed to provoke the eruption. Photoallergic lesions are typically raised little bumps that are red and papular. They appear on sun-exposed areas, such as the face, the "vee" of the neck, and the tops of the hands. If it's a bad case, they'll blister. They are most often caused by the following:

griseofulvin (an antibiotic used to treat fungal infections)
certain tetracyclines

hexachlorophene
water pills
certain oral diabetic medicines

4. *Purpuric Eruptions.* A purpuric eruption looks just like it sounds—like a purple bruise. They are not raised like a welt, but instead are flat areas of purple blotch located usually (though not always) on the extremities. The cause is a bleeding into the skin, most often as a reaction to one of the following:

Quinidine (a heart disease drug)
water pills
cortisone
barbiturates

5. *Blistering Reactions.* Blisters, filled either with blood or clear fluid, can show up anywhere on the body. The substances below are frequently associated with blister eruptions:

iodides (often in vitamin pills and naturally in shellfish and many health foods)
bromides
mercury
phenolphthalein (a common ingredient in laxatives, and also used as a coloring in cheap wine)
arsenic (formerly an ingredient in many Victorian-era tonics that replaced indoor pallor with a ruddy complexion)

6. *Pigmentary Changes.* Some drugs and medicines can cause skin either to lighten or darken, with or without sun exposure.

birth-control pills
arsenic

chloroquine (widely used as a prophylactic for malaria, this drug can cause pigmentary changes, most often on sun-exposed skin areas)

7. *Fixed Drug Eruptions.* These are allergic reactions that occur over and over on the very same spot. For example, every time you get a penicillin shot, you might get a cluster of purplish blisters on your left cheek. And every time it happens, the eruption might take longer to go away. The affected skin can also become steadily darker, and if the source of irritation isn't discontinued, what started as a pesky eruption can turn into an ugly bull's-eye. Our example of penicillin is not a common cause; much more so are:

birth-control pills
phenolphthalein
barbiturates
gold
sulfur drugs (including sulfonamides and antibiotics containing sulfur)

8. *Darkening at Injection Site.* It's not a frequent reaction, but iron injections will sometimes cause brown to blue discolorations where the needle entered the skin. These dark patches are unattractive and take considerable time to fade. Iron treatments are often prescribed for women who have become anemic following childbirth.

9. *Lichen Planus-like Eruptions.* The itchy violet papules of lichen planus were described in Chapter 4. Although they can show up anywhere on the body, this grouped papular eruption is most often seen on the wrists. Some drugs provoke a response in some individuals that isn't

lichen planus, but looks just like it. Drugs that can cause it include:

Dilantin
water pills
gold

10. *Ichthyosis.* Some patients suffer from dry skin and accentuated skin markings, especially on the lower extremities. This condition looks like fish scales, and it's sometimes a result of treatment with certain anticholesterol drugs. Nicotinic acid, another drug used mainly to treat vascular problems, is also associated with scaly skin. Some doctors prescribe nicotinic acid as an all-purpose pep-up in addition to its role in vascular disorders.

11. *Erythema Nodosum.* A painful condition of multiple large bumps on the fronts of the legs and/or forearms, this condition is a reaction noted most often among young women and can be accompanied by fever or arthritis. What unlucky allergy provokes an outbreak?

penicillin
codeine
sulfonamides

12. *Hair Loss.* Although not specifically an eruption, hair loss is nonetheless a very real and troublesome reaction to certain medications, such as:

birth-control pills
anticoagulants
certain cancer drugs

13. *Acne.* The following substances sometimes cause pustular reactions and/or acne-type eruptions:

cortisone
progesterone-type birth-control pills
iodides
bromides
INH (an anti-TB drug)

The Side Effects of Certain Commonly Used Drugs

Once again, I must reiterate that whether or not you have a reaction to any of the drugs, substances, or medicines noted in this chapter is strictly a matter of your own personal level of sensitization. The concept here is end organ sensitivity, which in this context refers to the variable tolerance levels of the end organ called your skin. Whether the presence of any medicine will sensitize you and lead to an allergic-type eruption is not automatically predictable. The reactions described below have been frequently noted, but they most certainly do not befall everybody.

Valium. It's quite rare to see a drug eruption stemming from this ubiquitous tranquilizer, but the pill has been reported to cause hives. However, the hives may well be triggered by the original nervousness instead of the Valium.

Aspirin. Aspirin decreases the clotting factor in your blood. And this can lead to black and blue marks almost anywhere on the body. These little bruises are not always easy to spot and sometimes aren't noticed at all. Aspirin can also trigger an eruption of hives in some people. It is interesting to note that the anticlotting effect of one aspirin will last up to two weeks.

Vitamins. The extra quantities of iodides and bromides that fortify many vitamin pills can cause acne. These two substances commonly cause pustular reactions in the skin.

Cortisone. This drug, widely prescribed to counter other allergic reactions, can become highly androgenic when metabolized. Androgens are closely related to acne outbreaks, and people on cortisone usually do get pimples.

Laxatives. When they contain phenolphthalein, as they often do, there is a chance of a fixed drug eruption.

Antibiotics. Penicillin can cause hives and generalized drug eruptions, sometimes fatally. These reactions are more common among allergic-type people and those with eczema. If this is you, have your doctor be extra sure you're not allergic to the drug before undergoing any treatment. This is especially true nowadays since the new long-acting injectable penicillin can stay in your system for weeks.

Ampicillin is a widely (some say overly) used antibiotic that causes bad drug eruptions in from 5 percent to 10 percent of patients. These eruptions characteristically get a little worse after you stop the medication. If you have mononucleosis, you run a particularly large risk of getting widespread, brick-red, rashes from Ampicillin.

Tetracycline, which is widely and wisely used for acne treatment, is usually quite safe. However, certain types, like Declomycin, are commonly associated with photo-eruptions in conjunction with sunlight. Additionally, the drug can also cause yeast infections in young women and occasionally hives.

Birth-Control Pills. What a wonder they are, and how fortunate it is that so many women can use them so safely. But among the unlucky, they can cause acne, hair loss, darkening of skin on the cheeks (chloasma), fixed drug eruptions, and hives!

Librium. Like Valium, this pill is occasionally connected with hives or generalized eruptions.

Chapter 14

Today's Techniques of Skin Restoration

You say your skin is hopelessly scored with deep wrinkles and sun-baked age lines? And everybody tells you that sun-damaged skin can never be repaired, right? Or perhaps your legacy from adolescent acne is pockmarks and acne scars. Take heart. Your skin can be rejuvenated, and in many cases you can get rid of those pocks or wrinkles.

It is true that sun can severely damage the skin, especially after many years of overexposure. However, the damage can definitely be repaired. When I biopsy a piece of sun-damaged tissue, what it shows me is elastosis. This is a degeneration of the elastic fibers in the dermis, and it's the cause of many wrinkles and sagging. If the damage is really severe, I can also note what's called "slight disorganization" in the epidermis. This means the cells are bigger than usual, and the connecting bridges between them are a little askew, so that they don't butt up properly against one another. The epidermis also varies unnaturally in thickness.

Slight disorganization causes those small cruddy places

where the skin is just messed up and never looks right. When disorganization is really severe, every cell breaks loose, goes its own way, and you have skin cancer. In Chapter 12 I described how skin cancer isn't the threat people traditionally expect "cancer" to be. At this point it is interesting to note that the very similarity of badly sun-damaged and precancerous skin is what allows a new miracle drug to treat them both so effectively without surgery.

Topical 5-Fluorouracil Ointment

This drug has amazing results when applied topically. The common brand names you'll hear are Efudex and Fluoroplex, both of which are available with a prescription and come in varying strengths. A potent antagonist to gastrointestinal and other internal cancers 5-fluorouracil has the same effect when applied to disorganized cells in the skin.

What 5-fluorouracil does is to selectively seek out and destroy disorganized tissue. Its major strength is that it not only safely destroys obviously damaged tissue, but it also seeks out tissue that looks fine now but will show damage in the next four or five years. You can use it anywhere on the body, and it can greatly improve looks while actually eliminating possible future skin cancers.

This is not the treatment for everyone with a skin problem. The typical person who would benefit most might be a fifty-year-old woman who has spent the last twenty-six winters on the beach in Barbados. Or the former navy man who baked his face to a crisp for three years in the South Pacific and looks terribly aged even though he hasn't been out in the sun for the last twenty years. Curiously, it also helps to have fair skin and light

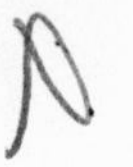

eyes; the ointment just seems to work better on these people.

Many doctors don't know about 5-fluorouracil, and those who do will use it only on patients they trust. For all its effectiveness, it's not the most pleasant treatment in the world. First, the ointment must be applied once a day for three to four weeks while the patient watches for red spots to develop. These spots occur not only on the heavy wrinkles and bad blotches, but also in areas you thought were perfectly healthy. Sometimes, a little sun exposure is recommended to hasten the process.

The red spots get redder and redder, finally begin to ooze, and sometimes ulcerate. At this point, the ointment is discontinued, and the treatment switches to anti-inflammation creams and cold-water compresses. It's rather like having bad poison ivy. Many patients hate it all so much, however, that they discontinue the ointment too early.

Gradually, the redness and oozing go away, usually over a period of four to six weeks, and new skin grows. After two months to ten weeks from the first application, some patients may look years younger. The treatment is mostly employed on people over forty, and in fact you can't be too old for it to work. The major drawback is cosmetic—it really makes you look horrible and is obviously not recommended for trial lawyers, salespeople, politicians, or anyone who works continually in the public eye.

Is it painful? No, not particularly. The effect is that of a contact dermatitis, whose rash is bothersome but not excruciating. It's thought that 5-fluorouracil actually makes you allergic to your own disorganized tissue. It's also been shown to have good results with psoriasis when nothing else works. And it's a help with psoriasis on the fingernails when injections into the nail itself are not possible. If you can bear with it, especially through the last four or five weeks, the treatment will literally give you a younger looking face or a nice new de-spotted pair of hands!

Chemabrasion

Sometimes pocks and/or wrinkles respond better to chemical peeling (chemabrasion). Your doctor has to decide whether this method is better than 5-fluorouracil. In general, I would describe the typical chemabrasion candidate as a forty-year-old woman or man with a proliferation of fine wrinkles around the eyes and lips or a twenty-five-year-old former acne sufferer whose acne has burnt out but left bad pocks and scars.

The treatment comprises application of highly irritating chemicals that literally burn off the top layers of skin. Trichloroacetic acid is most often used, sometimes in conjunction with (or occasionally substituted by) phenol and/or resorcinol. The process is not cheap, even though it seldom requires more than two back-to-back visits to the doctor's office.

In my office the first step is to evaluate the patient psychologically. Chemabrasion is no miraculous key to happiness, nor is it a second chance at life. An unstable patient with unreasonable expectations won't get a chemabrasion from me. Then there are the people who still have active acne, in which case the treatment is again not recommended. No point paying all that money if the source of the problem is active and liable to cause a recurrence. There's also a danger of post-inflammatory hyper- or hypopigmentation (darkening or lightening of the skin) for black or Mediterranean complexioned people. Under these circumstances the chemabrasion process is still possible, but it must be done with milder solutions and stringent warnings to the patient to *keep out of the sun.* Sometimes a trial run on a portion of the forearm is good insurance that the procedure won't do more damage than good.

The actual peeling process goes like this. I first give the patient five to ten milligrams of Valium, pull the hair back, and degrease the face with Seba-Nil (a good OTC astringent). The patient lies down, and the peeling agent, usually in gel form, is applied evenly to the face and left on for twenty minutes to half an hour. Gradually, a burning sensation becomes worse and worse; sometimes the patient will have to sit up in front of a fan if the pain becomes too uncomfortable. At the end of the treatment, the gel is washed off with water, leaving the skin whitish and not very attractive.

This whole procedure is repeated the following day. The skin's whitish color results from the precipitation of trichloroacetic acid in the presence of epidermal proteins. Were it not for this chemical reaction, the acid would burn through the skin like a blowtorch.

The patient keeps applying a mild lubricating lotion, stays out of the sun, and waits for the whitish skin to peel away in sheets, usually four to seven days after the first application, revealing the healthy growing tissue below. This unfortunately looks at first a little like raw liver, so most chemabrasion patients go into self-imposed exile. I like to encourage people not to be embarrassed. You were brave to get the treatment, and it often encourages friends who need it to get it too.

I said earlier that chemabrasion was no miracle, but I'll add here that it almost always results in some improvement. It's a rule of thumb that the worse the scars, the more remarkable the improvement. People with fair skin and light eyes will again show the best results.

Dermabrasion

This is another route many have followed to smooth new skin. The dermabrasion candidate has much in common with his/her chemabrasion counterpart, and in fact the two procedures are often used in concert. It's at the discretion of the dermatologist, who must evaluate the nature of the lines and/or pocks to be removed.

The process itself requires a dermabrader, which is a small hand-held machine with a diamond burr. The patient is given Valium or a similar tranquilizer, and the skin is degreased with an astringent. A skilled assistant is necessary to hold taut each portion of skin to be treated. First I mark the bottom of the line or pock with a purple dye. Next the skin is sprayed with an aerosol freezing spray. I'll go through ten cans of fluoroethyl spray on one patient, since it's necessary to freeze solid the area to be abraded. When the skin is rigid, I start abrading and continue until the purple color is gone.

This requires constant application of the freeze spray, diligent attention on the part of both dermatologist and assistant, and a good deal of endurance on the part of the patient. It's not the abrader that hurts so much, but the constant freezing of the skin. When the sanding down is completed, bandages are applied, under which crusts will quickly form. When the crusts fall off, they leave raw sensitive skin, which will eventually grow out considerably smoother than before.

To someone who started out badly pocked or scarred, it will literally look like magic. But there are certain problems to beware, most important of which is the danger that the doctor might go too far with the dermabrader. That can leave a scar worse than those the patient has come to have sanded away. The treatment is also bloody, rather painful, and considerably more expensive than chemabrasion. It is also widely sought by people who don't really need it.

Over-the-Counter Facials and Masks

Drugstores are filled with these pleasant smelling preparations. They make your face feel tingly and deeply cleaned. They promote a degree of peeling, but are simply not strong enough to really attack the problems of sun-damage lines or acne scars. "Peach Mask Melba" or whatever the latest facial confection is may feel great but should not be expected to alleviate any serious skin problems.

Silicone

Silicone is an inert chemical whose debut on the beauty scene some years back seemed like a dream come true. It's a filler, and when injected drop by drop along the length of an age line or scar, it will puff it out. However, there is a fine line between proper injection and overinjection. The latter causes an unattractive puffiness.

Silicone burst into prominence via breast implants. Until several years ago, it was medically impure, available only on the black market, and implants generally had to be obtained overseas. The problem that soon developed stemmed from the chemical's tendency to migrate around the body. Not only do lumps of silicone meander, but the body itself tends to form tissue around the wandering clumps in an attempt to entrap them. Increasing numbers of people had silicone rattling all around them; sometimes cancer resulted.

Nowadays, there is a new, safe silicone that is medically pure. Contained in a nonmigrating bag, it's implanted—bag and all—into the breasts only. At this writing it's the only legal form of silicone treatment in the United States. There is another type of silicone for injection into facial lines, but it is not yet approved by the Federal Drug Administration. Pending approval, ten doctors in the country have FDA permission to use it. It is known, however, that this treatment is offered illegally by people not approved by the FDA. So if you're searching for silicone injections of this nature, ask your doctor or the FDA to direct you to properly designated practitioners.

Will line injections receive FDA approval? For a while, it seemed certain; now it's not so sure; and I myself have no idea.

Chapter 15

Losing Your Hair?

Hair is a charlatan's game, and most people know so little about it that they fall easy prey to the most preposterous claims. Whereas most mammals depend on it for warmth, we humans no longer have any medical need for hair. It is an item of psychological adornment, symbolic of strength and youth. This potent symbolism explains the acute anxiety that's triggered by noticeable hair loss.

Hair growth, like the seasons, is cyclical. And every hair on your head (there are some 100,000 follicles on the "average" scalp) has its own timetable. There is an anagen (growth) phase that lasts anywhere from two to six (usually four) years. After that, the hair follicle stops growing hair and rests for about three months. After the rest period, called the telogen phase, growth begins again. But the old hair, which was always dead (only the follicle is alive), is actually pushed out by new hair produced by the reawakened follicle. Therefore, hair loss can be a good signal, since it often announces the beginning of a new anagen phase.

The follicles do not operate in concert fortunately; otherwise we would all go through total periodic baldness. At any given point, about 85 percent of the hair follicles on a healthy head will be in the anagen phase. Those that aren't will drop about 100 to 150 hairs per day, the normal rate.

Aristotle, who was bald himself, often wondered at the flowing tresses of the palace eunuchs. What he didn't know was that when their testicles went, so went their ability to produce the hormone androgen. Androgen causes hair loss, and it is your hair follicles' sensitivity to androgen that determines when and if it happens to you. The follicles on the crown of the head and those at the top of the forehead are most sensitive to androgens. Typical male pattern baldness, as it is called, starts in those regions, then gradually erodes the hair in between. Follicles at the side of the scalp are the hardiest and the last to go.

Like acne, hair loss is a matter of end organ sensitivity. It varies dramatically from person to person and is determined by heredity. If your parents have weak follicles, the chances are overwhelming that you'll fare similarly. It's amazing how much our physical development repeats that of our parents. Although baldness sometimes seems to skip generations, the gene is there somewhere, and there isn't much you can do about it except be stoic, get a wig, or have a hair transplant. Women are luckier than men in that female hair loss is seldom total. But it can be sufficient to cause significant cosmetic damage. This, in turn, leads both sexes to spend money on worthless hair preparations.

Hair is dead. When I talk about growth and rest phases, it's the follicle to which I'm referring. Located in the dermis layer of the skin, it is one of the most rapidly metabolizing organs in the body and is highly sensitive to changes in diet or in the nervous system. Our follicles will proceed on their aforementioned schedule (except for eyebrows and lashes, which grow for ten weeks, then rest for nine months) unless disturbed. Curiously, hair falls out when the leaves fall. This would seem to indicate at least an unconscious identification with the rhythms of the natural world. Hair also falls out after extraordinary physical or psychological traumas. Major shocks—a death in the family, being hit by a bus—will throw hair follicles into the telogen phase. You've heard of hair turning white overnight? Well, it doesn't quite happen overnight. But hair can be thrown abruptly and totally into the telogen phase by some shock, then all fall out. When the anagen phase begins again, the new hairs can grow in without coloration.

The prime cause of baldness is the gradually accumulating levels of androgen that result from maturation of the adult body. When the blood level of androgen reaches a critical level, the follicles are put to sleep (the most sensitive first). Hair follicles actually are very hard to kill, and nearly all of them retain their ability to grow hair even on heads that are bald as the proverbial billiard ball. If one could inject an androgen antagonist into a hair follicle on your Uncle Charlie's bald head, a hair would probably grow. Unfortunately, this treatment might also give Uncle Charlie cancer, which is why it is not practiced. Every drug and cosmetic company in the country is working on a solution to this, so we may actually see a day soon when hair follicles can be safely stimulated.

How much hair can you lose before the thinning becomes noticeable? The answer is about 10 percent. People who hit this level will often rush to an exotic hair treatment salon, where they can lose their money as fast as their hair. These slick establishments, with their fancy

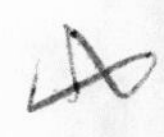

lobbies and complimentary glasses of wine, are masterworks of theatrical staging. The patron typically undergoes shampoos, scalp massage, application of tincture of capsicum (this is only pepper, and it makes the scalp tingle), sunlamp treatment, and a competent blow-dry. After all this, you'll look better (temporarily) and feel like things have really happened. But whether any of this really affects hair loss is highly questionable.

The scalp has the heaviest web of blood vessels anywhere in the body, which is why head wounds are always so bloody. The suggestion that salon massages or sunlamp treatments increase blood flow and/or ameliorate hair loss is simply not true. These salons do nothing for the hair follicle, which is the critical organ of hair production and loss.

Dandruff, those dry white flakes that accumulate between washings and sometimes itch, is normally caused by a mild increase in the shedding rate of epidermal cells on the scalp. It doesn't cause hair loss, since it is unrelated to hair follicles, which are in the dermis. Sometimes, however, dandruff isn't really dandruff. It might be psoriasis of the scalp or eczema or even nits. Nits often plague people each spring after the warm weather sets in. What happens is a person will stretch out on a lawn somewhere, and small mites will crawl into the hair and lay eggs. Nits cluster around the hair shaft, while dandruff lies on the scalp. Then there are pseudo-nits that look just like the genuine article but are actually accumulated bits of hair spray!

The various treatments for these conditions are well established. Topical steroids will abate eczema and psoriasis. Doctors kill nits with various chemicals. And pseudo-nits are eliminated when you stop using hair spray. Dandruff should be treated by a variety of easily available shampoos. I say variety since the condition seems to react more favorably when more than one shampoo is used. I advise that you buy a selection of products that each utilizes a different active ingredient. If you alternate between Head & Shoulders (which contains zinc pyrithione), Selsun (with selenium sulfide), Zetar (or any of the other tar-base shampoos), and Sebulex (a peeling shampoo), you will more effectively counter the dandruff than if you were to stick with any one product exclusively. Sunlight, incidentally, is very good for dandruff sufferers.

I'm afraid that natural baldness can only be laid at the twin doorsteps of androgen and old age. As we grow older the follicles will atrophy and gradually lose their ability to produce hair. At the same time, the melanocytes will experience similar atrophy and lose their ability to produce pigment. So the hair that still grows becomes gray.

Of course, there is a chance that some medical problem is causing you to lose your hair. Hair loss can be a symptom of both anemia and thyroid disease and it is reversible when these conditions are diagnosed and treated properly. Undue and/or unremitting stress can also throw an otherwise healthy head of hair into the telogen phase. If the anxiety continues without relief, the anagen (growth) phase can be postponed indefinitely while the remaining hairs fall out.

Sometimes people are taking medication that is causing hair loss. Hormone shots that induce the female period are a case in point. These androgen and androgen-related hormones can have the same effect if they play a large part in the diet.

Cessation of estrogen-type birth-control pills can result in sudden hair loss. Stop the pill, reduce estrogen levels in the body, and hair loss is frequently the result. Menopause has the same effect, since it signals significant lessening of the amount of estrogen produced by the woman's body.

If none of this applies to you, and you still feel your hair loss is excessive, maybe you are suffering from trichotilomania, a stress-related condition described in Chapter 4. In that case, you're so nervous you're pulling your own hair out without even realizing it. A typical symptom of this condition is a hot denial that you could possibly have it.

If you're not pulling out your hair unconsciously, maybe you're doing it consciously! Pulled-back ponytail-type hairstyles actually exert enough pressure on hair follicles to kill them. This is worth noting, since it is one of the few conditions that will actually permanently disable a hair follicle. Many women straighten their hair with hot oils too. This can cause what's called hot-comb alopecia, in which you essentially fry your own follicles. Result: hair loss.

If you think you might be losing your hair too fast, the first thing you can do each day is count it. Don't laugh, lots of people do! Of course, the hairs to count are the ones that are falling out. Do it on days when you don't shampoo, and never in the fall when hair tends to fall out anyway. Brush three times daily and count the hairs that come out on the brush. If it's between 100 and 150 hairs a day, you're OK.

Alternately, you can ask your doctor to administer any of a number of well-established tests that will tell you whether your hair loss problem is treatable or not.

First, you should get a CBC (complete blood count). The purpose of this is to find out whether you're anemic (malnutrition stops hair growth). Most people who are were very surprised to discover it. Maybe anemia is your problem too. The CBC can be normal, however, and you can still have a subclinical iron deficiency. So, you should also get a serum iron test and an iron binding capacity test. These will ascertain the levels of iron in your system, which, if deficient, can be easily supplemented by shots or pills. Not always, but sometimes, big doses of iron will make hair grow. At least in iron deficient people.

If your thyroid's on the blink, it can be easily determined by a pair of tests called T-3 and T-4. If the thyroid level in the blood is unbalanced—either too much or too little—it can cause undue hair loss. Finally, women can quite simply determine whether they are estrogen deficient. Your gynecologist can tell you by means of a smear test of the cervix. If you are deficient, hormone treatments or sometimes just a change to estrogen-type birth-control pills will be enough to reverse a potentially frightening rate of hair fallout.

However, if you pass all these tests with flying colors, have no serious systemic disease, and are still losing your hair, then my advice is either to resign yourself gracefully or resort to non-medical means. By that, I mean surgery and hair transplants (see Chapter 16). For now, I want to comfort you with the knowledge that hair transplants are always a last resort, and they really work quite well. Don't be too hasty in your reactions to natural hair loss. Statistical odds favor you to keep almost all of what you've got at age thirty. If you're not there yet, wait; if you are, don't decide on a radical treatment based on hair loss in the mid to late twenties. Hair loss comes in waves, and there can be long stretches in between.

Thinning hair also afflicts those who are neither anemic, under stress, shot full of hormones, nor ancient with age. Acute schizophrenia, depression, or anxiety will throw the hair much more massively into the telogen phase than everyday stress. Similarly, a three-week coma after, say, a collision with a diesel train will cause the same thing. It's called telogen effluvium, in the trade, a

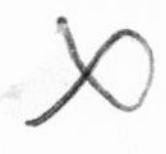

massive conversion of otherwise healthy hair into the non-growth telogen phase resulting from trauma. Some medicines cause telogen effluvium, most notably heparin and coumadin, both used to treat clot patients.

Hair loss can tell you things about yourself too. In addition to being a symptom of anemia and thyroid conditions, it is also symptomatic of more exotic situations. Thallium, which is rat poison, causes hair loss in humans. So does mercury (from polluted fish), lead (from paint), and arsenic (from old ladies and lace).

Certain dermatological conditions include hair loss as a side effect. Generalized eczema wreaks havoc with hair follicles, as does skin cancer, fungal infections, and acute psoriasis. Secondary syphilis results in what's called the moth-eaten pattern of baldness, which is characterized by small, scattered bald patches. Bigger bald patches are seen in the condition called alopecia areata, wherein the sufferer strangely enough is thought to become allergic to his or her own hair. This is commonly related to stress and/or anemia and is usually treated with steroid injections to the affected areas. The steroids will usually reverse the process. Finally, when certain nerve diseases, like lichen planus, occur on the scalp, they will kill the hair follicles. Fortunately, they rarely occur there.

To minimize the effect of genetically determined hair loss:

1. Eat a well-balanced diet, avoid androgenic foods (wheat germ, liver, etc.), and watch out for freaky vitamin-deficient diets. You can also take iron supplements, which sometimes help women, occasionally help men, and don't hurt anybody.

2. Find a good shampoo, preferably one with protein. Shampooing really has nothing to do with hair loss, but protein coats the hair fiber and makes it look thicker. It's contained in many shampoos and conditioners, as well as

in certain products that do nothing but give a thickened appearance. If your hair tends to be oily, shampoo more often; if it's really oily, use soap. If you have dry hair, don't shampoo so often. And don't worry about the hair that comes out in the wash. It's only telogen hair that would have come out tomorrow or the next day. Even excess shampooing will not cause accelerated hair loss.

3. Get a good hair stylist. Blow-drying won't hurt you, unless you burn the scalp. Neither will brushes, despite the claims of certain manufacturers.

4. Avoid stress and be calm with the knowledge that you can always have a hair transplant that will probably fix you up amazingly well. Alternately, in a few more years some young genius will very possibly have discovered a way to safely stimulate fallow follicles. A lot of smart minds are working on exactly this problem, so we'll all wait and see.

Chapter 16

Transplants, Implants, Hairweaves, and Wigs

Hair loss does not discriminate on the basis of sex. So what's called male pattern baldness—the gradual recession of the hairline to meet a gradually growing bald spot on the crown—can just as well happen to women. It's hereditary, so there's nothing you can do to stop it! Women, though, suffer to a lesser degree than men.

Sometimes people lose their hair for reasons other than genes. Chapter 15 describes the most common causes of unnecessary hair loss. We're directing our attention now to those hair follicles, usually on the top of the head, whose sensitivity to the hormone androgen in the blood gradually renders them dormant.

The crux of balding is, once again, end organ sensitivity. Hair follicles (the end organs in question) are completely different on top of the head than they are along the sides. The degree of resilience among variously located follicles, as I say, is a matter of genes. There's no special formula for prognostication; baldness isn't accurately forecast by noting the scalp of one's maternal grandfather for instance. Genes for strong follicles are shuffled among parents and families, and either you have them or you don't. Your parents are usually, though not always, the most accurate indication of your own future appearance.

If you are losing your hair and want to do something about it, don't despair. The cosmetic appearance of a full head of hair is well within reach, and you have several well-tested options from which to choose. In fact, I take special pains to emphasize this point. Often the knowledge that reliable solutions are available for use at any time will deter premature application of these same remedies. For instance, someone who's twenty years of age, has no genetic history of baldness, and who's still losing his or her hair, should probably wait and do nothing. Hair loss comes in spurts, and it's often temporary. The follicles themselves rarely die, and though they may temporarily stop producing hair, they will often start again too. Even if the hair loss is permanent, twenty is too young for the situation to be stabilized. A front area transplant, for instance, might become stranded by continuing recession of the hairline.

Age twenty-five is about the youngest to consider a transplant or implant. And it's better to wait until thirty, when the hairline is almost always stabilized. If you want a transplant then, fine; but by all means don't rush into it when you're eighteen!

Hair Transplants

This technique is extremely successful, employed widely by both sexes (however, more common in males), and doesn't hurt all that much. Healthy androgen-resistant follicles are simply taken from areas along the sides of the scalp and planted, like so many geraniums, on the top, or wherever necessary.

Many people really don't need a transplant. I frequently counsel people to do nothing and be peaceful. But other times the cosmetic appeal is irresistible. And, of course, there are instances of bad scars or burns on the head that transplants will hide completely.

This is how it's done. Your doctor will lift a layer of hair at the back or side of the scalp and shave a small area of these less-sensitive (to androgen) follicles. The lifted layer of hair will later cover this area completely. Next, a local anesthetic is injected (usually a shot of Xylocaine with epinephrine), followed by a freeze spray. This procedure numbs the skin, and the epinephrine helps constrict blood vessels. This is important, since the head is richly supplied with blood, and head operations of any sort are liable to be bloody. This bloodiness, even though it is neither serious nor particularly dangerous, has caused many a two-hundred-pound man to faint dead away! It happens quite often and is no cause for embarrassment.

When the healthy follicle area is prepared, the doctor will remove small shallow cylinders of flesh containing from eight to ten follicles apiece by means of a "transplant punch." This is a simple stainless steel tool whose sharp circular end is pressed against the skin and revolved by hand. It cuts little 3.5 millimeter circles called "plugs"; the cut goes right through the epidermis, the dermis, and into the fatty tissue below. After each plug is described into the flesh, the doctor will remove them all with a forceps and place them in a sterile saline solution. This keeps them fresh while the destination area is being prepared and while the fat is being carefully trimmed from the bottom of each plug.

How many plugs does the doctor cut? This is a matter of differing opinion. It's quite unbelievable how many plugs you can get out of the rim (alongside the scalp) without noticeable damage. Besides which, the process isn't pleasant, and I don't like to do less than fifty plugs at a time. Some doctors and patients prefer to start out with half that many and see how they grow. The point, however, is that the removal of fifty plugs at once is actually not much more work than a twenty-five-plug job. The price is usually by the plug, plus a fee for each visit to the doctor's office.

The number of plugs is also determined by the size and location of the bald area. These procedures typically require a number of visits, with rest periods in between to allow the transplanted hair to take root. Especially in the front—you can't expect to fill in an area 100 percent in one operation. Different patients have differing expectations as well. The transplanted hair that thrills one will still be too sparse for another.

The trimming of the fatty ends on each plug is a most important step. Usually the plugs come right out of the scalp and a scissor isn't necessary. But when the fat is trimmed, whoever does it must take pains not to injure the follicle roots. If possible the doctor should do his own trimming, and unless your doctor's assistant is unusually talented, you should expect him to do the same. Trimming also provides an opportunity to study the angle of hair growth, so that each plug can be positioned properly in its new location.

When the plugs are prepared, the bald area is anesthetized and the transplant punch is used to make receptacles. Some doctors take the receptacle plugs and insert them along the rim, but this isn't really necessary. However, it is necessary to space the receptacles in the transplant area about 3.5 millimeters apart. Whereas the rim area is covered with a layer of hair, the bald area will need enough healthy tissue between the receptacles to insure good blood nutrition. This lets the transplanted plugs take root in healthy tissue. A large number of plugs too close together can result in a necrosis of the scalp, where the tissue becomes black and infected.

When the trimmed plugs are inserted and aligned to grow in the right direction, no sutures are required. The plugs fit snugly and stay in of their own accord. Sometimes there's a little persistent bleeding, but even that usually goes away quickly, making a light bandage optional.

What happens next? The transplanted hair all falls out! The follicles have quite naturally been traumatized and thrown into the telogen phase (a temporary dormancy described in Chapter 15). Three months later hair starts to grow again, and it grows ferociously. In about two more months, the patient will typically return for another transplant to fill in the gaps between the now healthy transplanted hair. These gaps are more noticeable in the front, which usually dictates at least one and often more return visits. Transplants in the rear can sometimes be done to the patient's satisfaction in one visit.

Even though a transplant is not necessary to maintain the health of an individual, it is of psychological value just to know of its existence. The ideal patient is one who is about thirty years old, has a good rim, and a limited and well-defined area of baldness. Postoperative care is simple; the patient need only refrain from heavy exercise and shampoos for about a week and maybe wear a hat. After a week or two, it's hard to tell that an operation was even performed.

In good hands, almost every plug—95 out of 100—will take. It's amazing how well the treatment works. But patience is a prerequisite. A bald crown might take anywhere from several hundred to several thousand plugs—you might have to undergo surgery every six months for years. It depends on your expectations and at what level you're happy. The cost is not cheap, typically $7.50 to $15 per plug, plus a separate charge for each office visit.

Hair Implants

Hair implanting is a totally different technique. What the doctor does is take Teflon-covered staples and insert them into the scalp. A clump of either artificial or human hair is threaded through each staple, which is then driven down into the scalp with a gun.

The advantages are numerous. The hair replacement is immediate and, barring physical reactions, it's permanent. Implants also lend themselves to move extensive bald areas and are significantly cheaper than transplants.

My objection to this technique is the insertion of foreign bodies into the scalp. These staples come in a hundred varieties, and the Teflon-coating certainly minimizes tissue irritation. Still, many people get what's called "foreign body granuloma," in which irritated tissue will expel the staples. On the other hand, more people are able to tolerate the treatment well than not.

If you do have an implant, go to a doctor. While many salons and hair treatment centers offer implants, my feeling is that the mere possibility of complications requires a doctor's attention from the onset. And if you're black, be extra careful. You run a chance of developing keloidal scars.

Hairweaves

This method is as complex and tedious as it is popular. A hairweave requires the threading of your existing hairs through a nylon lattice until it sits flush on the scalp. It is then tied in place by knotting the hairs that pass through it. Once firmly anchored, the lattice is then woven with real or artificial hair until the affected area is covered completely.

Well, there are many things to recommend this procedure. It is safe and painless and threatens no physical reactions. But whereas the initial cost is a fraction of the hair transplant bill, the upkeep is endless and eventually quite expensive. After every few months of normal hair growth, you must return to the salon and have the lattice untied, moved down, and re-knotted at scalp level. Thus, you have a sort of maintenance monster. It can be worth it, however, especially because of the danger of keloidal scarring among the black men and women who comprise a sizable portion of the hairweave market.

Wigs

Of course, wigs predated all these treatments and have been a standby for centuries. On some people, they are actually undetectable. Unfortunately, on most people they are highly detectable, as well as being hot, uncomfortable, and expensive. Nobody has just one wig; you have to have two at least. And they have to be changed every year since the colors gradually oxidize and the hairs fall out.

Since transplants, implants, hairweaves, and wigs are not considered essential to good health, you are not allowed to take their considerable cost as a tax deduction. The only exception to this rule is when they obscure a disfiguring scar.

But there's an even more compelling reason for delay. Remember that the follicle never dies and never loses its ability to grow hair. I feel that it's simply a matter of time before some safe method is found to stimulate the follicles. Perhaps it will be an estrogen-like substance that combats the androgen effect; perhaps it will be some substance that slows the hair follicle's metabolism of androgen; perhaps it will be something utterly unheard of.

At this writing, there is nothing around that is FDA-approved. But it's my guess that within five to ten years some safe preparation will be on the market that you can literally rub on and grow hair!

Chapter 17

All You Ever Wanted to Know About Nails

Nail trouble is not only difficult to solve, it also usually signals worse trouble somewhere inside you. Your nails, like your eyes, are windows into the body. A doctor can look into a patient's eyes and tell, for example, whether he or she has high blood pressure or heart trouble. Likewise, nails (and hair too) are closely attuned to the general health of the body and can reflect anything from thyroid disease to a vitamin deficiency. Treatments for bad nails usually include programs of systemic medication (pills or medicines taken orally), painful injections into the nail bed sometimes, and lots of patience always.

Fingernails and toenails used to have more important functions than they do today. They once provided the human animal with protection for finger and toe tips, plus extra ability to grasp small objects. But like hair, our present existence requires only that they be cosmetically attractive.

Nail growth is quite variable. Believe it or not, your fingernails grow faster than your toenails, and nails on the same hand or foot will each grow at different rates.

(The average growth rate of a healthy nail is .1 millimeter per day.) Good nails are produced by the healthy skin that surrounds them; the nail itself is essentially dead. That's why ointments have little effect when applied directly to the nail.

Nails grow fastest on persons in their teens, and everybody's nails will grow faster in the summer than in the winter. Pregnancy speeds up nail growth, as does trauma (a bang with a hammer) and the regrowth following complete loss of a nail. Nail-biting will stimulate an increased growth rate, much the way pruning encourages a shrub. On the other hand, acute illness or starvation (actual or induced by crash dieting) will cause a growth slowdown.

The fact that nails are protein substances has given rise to a widely held misconception that they can be strengthened by eating gelatin. The gelatin theory has never been proved, and I don't believe it affects your nails at all. Iron pills, however, often cure iron-deficient people of the bad nails that typify that condition. (You might be iron deficient and not even know it. Easy to find out with a blood test.)

All Nails Are Divided into Three Parts

First there's the nail itself. Second is the nail fold, or skin that surrounds and borders on the nail itself. Third is the nail bed, the flesh that lies beneath each nail. Nail folds and nail beds are particularly subject to all manner of vicissitudes.

Nail Folds. Many people suffer from inflammation of the nail folds. It's a red swelling of the tissue bordering the nail itself and we've all seen it. Three of the most common causes are:

1. Inflammation resulting from the spread of disease from another part of the hand to the nail-producing skin that adjoins the nail itself. This is the simplest explanation.

2. Irritation from soaps and detergents. Most people think right away of the housewife stereotype with dishpan hands. But, in fact, many people of both sexes work with wet hands and sometimes irritating chemicals. Many people chronically wash their hands, too, and achieve the same inflammation.

3. Bartenders' Fingers. The medical term is paronychia, and it refers to the legion of bacteria, yeast, and fungus infections that can plague people who work with wet hands all day. Bartenders are particularly troubled because of the yeast, which is everywhere, including the beer that's forever all over their fingers.

If you've got, or are getting, this problem, I advise you to start making a point of keeping your fingers dry. Bad paronychia is not only painful, it also causes misshapen nails. Sometimes wearing rubber gloves is worth the protection. Sometimes application of an over-the-counter antibacterial ointment, like Bacitracin, will avert or abate bacterial infection. Bacitracin is good, since so many cases of paronychia do stem from bacteria, at least in part. But the causes can be multiple (yeast and/or fungus and/or bacteria). If you've really got it bad, go to a doctor who can prescribe an appropriate systemic medicine in addition to the suggestions above.

Nail Beds. Two common phenomena are associated with the nail beds: separation of the nail from the bed, and hemorrhages beneath the nail *in situ.* Here's the how and why of both:

Onycholysis is the medical term for the separation, to varying extents, of the nail from the skin beneath it. Whenever it happens, it's a setup for infection.

A traumatic bang from the hammer that missed the nail is a frequent cause. In fact, any consistent banging of the nail—and sometimes it's just an occupational hazard—will usually cause some separation. So will nail flickers' tick, which is a nervous habit of flicking the nails in succession with the thumbnail. Most of the time people do it unconsciously or with the semiconscious awareness of a tooth gnasher.

There can be systemic chemical reasons too, for example, medicines in your blood. The tetracycline so often prescribed for acne often causes phototoxic reactions when the patient goes out into the sun. Sufficient sunlight on the nails of someone taking tetracycline can cause the nails to separate badly or even fall off altogether. The sun can also be the catalyst for certain allergic reactions. You can have a contact allergy reaction to a certain nail lacquer or hardener that will cause your nails to fall off. Of course, most people don't have these reactions to nail products. Finally, hyper- or hypothyroid disease (too much or too little thyroid in the system) also causes nail separation.

Hemorrhages are the other major affliction of the nail bed. They appear as little red streaks of blood, usually near the tip of the nail. They sometimes result from the same things that cause onycholysis, particularly traumatic bangs and nail flickers' tick. But nail hemorrhages are also early symptoms of serious diseases, such as scurvy, liver disease, and trichinosis (from undercooked pork), to name only a few.

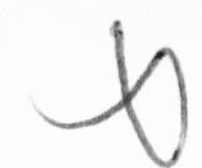

Common Skin Diseases and What They Do to Nails

Nails grow out of the skin, and their degree of health reflects the health of the skin they grow from. If the skin is afflicted from any of the conditions below, the nails will suffer too.

Psoriasis. This disease can often show up in the nails before it appears anywhere else on the body. The symptoms are oil spotting, which looks like it's under the nail, and hundreds of little pits on the nail surfaces.

Alopecia Areata. Also frequently stress-related (see Chapter 4), this is a condition in which the patient becomes temporarily allergic to his or her own hair. The observable symptoms include the appearance of small bald patches scattered around the scalp and hundreds of little pits in the nails.

Norwegian Scabies. This is a disease that's discussed at more length in Chapter 9. Basically, it's caused by an infestation of mites that crawl in under the nails as easily as anywhere else. The result is itching, and papules, and mite eggs between the fingers. The disease itself is very common, even though specific nail involvement is not. When it does affect the nails, it causes thickening, yellowing, and general uglification. Why Norwegian? Because the syndrome was first described from observations in a Norwegian old-age home.

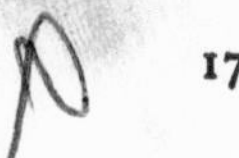

Body Secrets Your Nails Reveal

I said earlier that nails were windows into the body. Here is a list of the most commonly observed nail symptoms and a brief explanation of what they can tell you about yourself.

Whitening. The whole nail can become white because of a protein-deficient diet. In addition to poor nutrition, whitening nails are common symptoms of cirrhosis of the liver and kidney disease.

Separation of the Nails. A hyper- or hypothyroid condition will cause this, as will certain contact allergies to nail polishes and hardeners. Most women are not allergic to the polishes and hardeners on the market. As long as they keep the polish off the nail fold, there's usually not much to worry about. However, significant numbers do have allergic reactions, which result in nail separation.

Spooning. Concaving of the nail usually signals an iron deficiency, and happens especially—though not exclusively—to women.

Brittleness. Sometimes this results from arthritis. It's actually a thinning of the nail itself and is primarily a result of poor circulation.

Pigmentation. Your nails can turn a host of different colors for just as many reasons. Black nails are sometimes caused by surface application of topical ammoniated mercury, contained in many psoriasis products. Sometimes the nails are colored black by hair dyes, fungus infections, and photographic developers. Sometimes, a black nail can signify a cancerous tumor on the nail. Quite often, black nails are a symptom of vitamin B_{12} deficiency.

White horizontal bands on the nails are a symptom of arsenic or heavy metal (like mercury or silver) poisoning.

Blue-brown colored nails are caused by certain anti-malarial drugs. This is more common than you might think; Vietnam veterans and international pilots are both examples of groups who often take this medication. It discolors the hair too, but once the drug is discontinued, the symptoms abate.

Red-brown discolorations are usually the result of certain nail lacquers that oxidize the nail as they dry. The resorcinol in many acne products can cause the same discoloration.

Yes, you can even get green nails, from what's called a pseudomonas infection. This is a bacteria that loves wet fingers, especially those on nurses and bartenders.

What's Good for Your Nails?

If your nails are in poor condition, look at the circumstances of your life and use the information in this chapter to pinpoint the problem. Are you submitting them to constant traumas? Are you missing proper nourishment, because of chronic crash diets or vitamin B_{12} or C deficiencies? Did you buy a new nail cosmetic that's causing a contact allergy? Discover the problem first.

Having good nails is really so easy. Although most nail cosmetics won't hurt you, it's better to lay off and let the nail breathe. Keep the nails and fingers dry to avoid infection. Eat a balanced diet, possibly supplemented with vitamin C (helps combat hemorrhages) and/or iron (to prevent brittleness). Remember that gelatin does no good. Finally, don't overcut your nails and always make a rounded cut. Overcutting stimulates excessive growth. And square edges bite into nail folds to create the sort of little crannies that bacteria just love. If your nails get ingrown from bad shoes or awkward cuts, you might apply a little Bacitracin antibacterial ointment to safeguard against potential infection.

A Tip for Self-Diagnosis

Is that discoloration *on* your nail or under it? Easy to tell if you take a sharp knife and scrape the nail. If the shavings are colored, the discoloration is on top, and it's probably not very serious. If the shavings are white, then the problem's down below and is probably more serious than you thought.

A Bit of First Aid

Everybody's banged a nail and watched it painfully turn black. This is nothing but bleeding under the nail, and the pain results mostly from the pressure of the trapped fluid. Here's a painless way to relieve the pressure. Unravel a paper clip and heat one end red hot in a flame. You can push the heated end easily into the nail; it burns right through without punching. The fluid drains through the hole and relieves the pain. Your doctor can do this for you.

INDEX